Just Say Yes

Tenth Anniversary Edition

Just Say Yes
a marijuana memoir

Tenth Anniversary Edition

Catherine Hiller

Heliotrope Books
New York

Versions of these chapters were reprinted in Huffington Post from the following:

Chapter 1 Merry Jane, Snoop Dog's newsletter

Chapter 5 Purple Clover

Chapter 10 Green Flower Media

Chapter 12 Green Flower Media

Chapter 15 Green Flower Media

Chapter 16 MerryJane

A version of Chapter 3 was first published in *Honeysuckle* magazine (Winter 2018) as "Cannabis Thought Experiment."

A version of Chapter 6 was first published in the *New York Times* March 22, 2015 as "How I Buy Weed."

A version of Chapter 35 was first published in the anthology *Woodstock Revisited,* edited by Susan Reynolds (Adams Media, 2009) as "With the Film Crew."

Cover design by Judy Tipton-Katzman

Typeset by Naomi Rosenblatt

I have for many months hesitated about the propriety of allowing this, or any part of my narrative, to come before the public eye…and it is not without an anxious review of the reasons, for and against this step, that I have, at last, concluded on taking it.

—Thomas De Quincey
Confessions of an English Opium Eater, 1821

A writer without controversy is not a good one. A book without controversy is not a good one, either.

— Mo Yan
Winner, Nobel Prize for Literature, 2012

To Sonia

Table of Contents

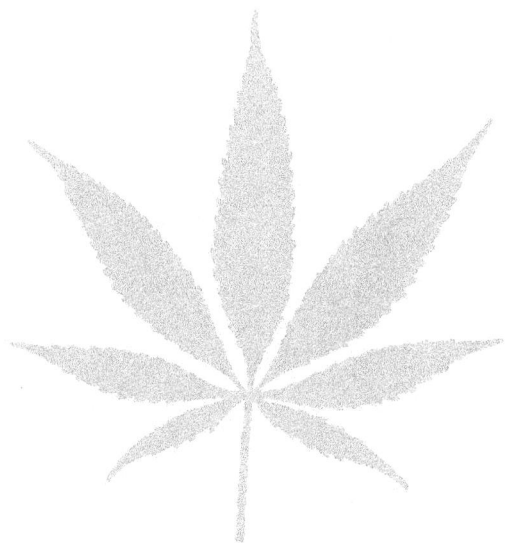

Foreword to the Tenth Anniversary Edition of *Just Say Yes*

This is the second edition of *Just Say Yes*.

The first edition was released in 2015 and it dropped like a bomb. One of the first public accounts of personal cannabis use by a respected East Coast professional, this charming little book exploded the stereotype of the lazy stoner. Especially after the *New York Times* decided to publish much of the first chapter as an Op-Ed.

Catherine Hiller's carefully concealed half century of cannabis consumption was suddenly exposed to the world, including her colleagues and Westchester neighbors. Millions of people learned how she had navigated her most important life passages—college, dating, marriage, motherhood, career, divorce, and deaths—with cannabis as a steadfast friend, almost always by her side. Hiller's successful trajectory through life stood out as a living rebuke to the old prohibitionist myths that cannabis use leads inexorably to addiction, psychosis, and moral decline.

The *Times* publication kicked off weeks of interviews in smaller media outlets: radio and tv stations, local newspapers, and podcasts. Hiller's stance throughout was that of a committed cannabis consumer—and of a self-described suburban housewife (although she has written several novels). She didn't shy away from the difficult questions; her tone was accessible, and her background and lifestyle endowed her with broad mainstream credibility.

It was the beginning of a widespread reconsideration of cannabis in the state and city of New York.

The landscape of cannabis has changed dramatically in the ten years since then. The number of states that have fully legalized has grown from four to twenty-four, and the number of medical states has climbed from twenty-three to thirty-eight. The amount of legal cannabis sales nationwide has increased from $5.4 Billion to $33.6 Billion annually, and the taxes collected on those sales have climbed from $135 million to $4 billion.

The growth in revenue and taxes is mirrored in the growth of cannabis employment. In 2015, there weren't even any figures available about the number of people employed in the new legal industry. The first estimates available for legal cannabis employment came out in 2017, and put the number at around 200,000 part- and full-time jobs. Today at least 417,000 people have found full time employment in the cannabis industry—about the same number working in beverage or apparel manufacturing, and orders of magnitude larger than coal mining.

Many of these newly employed workers are now in New York. Hiller's home state legalized cannabis in March of 2021, and issued its first cultivation and dispensary licenses in 2022.

The new industry has been gearing up since then; the first legal crops have been harvested, retailers have opened their doors, and millions of New Yorkers have legal access to cannabis for the first time in their lives.

New York's law is notable in several regards. It gave licensing priority to people with cannabis convictions, to those who lived in neighborhoods disproportionately harmed by cannabis prohibition, and to community-based organizations. Some of my friends who served time for cannabis in New York prisons now have licenses to practice their profession legally. The number of arrests for cannabis possession have dropped from forty thousand to less than one hundred—and it is legal to smoke a joint anywhere in the state that it is legal to smoke a cigarette.

Part of the fun of reading *Just Say Yes* today is appreciating just how much the landscape of cannabis has changed; of understanding that many of the vignettes so beautifully portrayed in the book are rapidly becoming things of the past: the logistics and etiquette of scoring weed from an underground dealer, the precautions taken to carry cannabis without getting busted, the glossary of code words, the search for a safe places to sneak a smoke; the multifold techniques to properly conceal a stash; the time-proven methods to conceal the signs of recent cannabis consumption.

Another part of the fun is the structure of the book itself. Hiller unspools her lifelong love affair with cannabis in reverse chronology; so lyrically, so deftly and smoothly you almost don't notice she is playing with you, that the movie is actually running backwards. She artfully portrays the timeless joys of consuming cannabis: the accelerated bonding that flows from sharing cannabis, the unique pleasure of cannabis infused conversations; the way cannabis can put us in closer touch with nature, with ourselves, with our children, and even with our parents.

Hiller's advocacy is gentle but nonetheless insistent. She packs a solid core of serious argument inside her pillow of mainstream accessibility. She lays out the hard realities of the racist origins of cannabis prohibition and the injustice of cannabis enforcement today. Again and again, she reminds readers that even as their rights may be expanding, tens of thousands of people in the United States remain in prison for non-violent cannabis convictions. None of them are criminals; they are our heroes, heroes who carried this healing plant through the darkness of Prohibition. We must bring them all home.

I invite you to enjoy *Just Say Yes*, and then let it be a call to action. May each of us do all we can to ensure that the benefits of change are shared by all, and that the shadows of the past no longer shackle our future.

✳ Steve DeAngelo is a lifelong cannabis activist,
                                entrepreneur, and author

1
Coming Out Green

In March, 2015, I came out green to two million people: the circulation of the Sunday *New York Times*.

I hadn't expected to come out in such a spectacular fashion—in the most public way imaginable. True, I was about to publish *Just Say Yes: A Marijuana Memoir*, in which I was frank and enthusiastic about my longtime cannabis use. Candor was the point: it never occurred to me to use a pseudonym. But most memoirs published by small, independent presses like mine sell just a few hundred copies, and most are reviewed only on blogs or on Amazon.

My expectations were not as high as I was when I wrote the memoir!

I enjoyed writing the book because of the two challenges it posed: first, how to use cannabis as a spine for the important events in my life, and, second, how to infuse the book with momentum while going backward in time. Each chapter starts at an earlier point than the one before, so the book begins in the present and ends when I'm a little girl, spinning to get dizzy and collapse. These narrative strategies distracted me from worrying about how much I was exposing myself to my readers. My basic assumption was that a couple of hundred strangers would read my little paean to pot—as well as my close friends and relations, who already know about my predilection.

I did not expect that over the course of three days in March, editing clients, distant acquaintances, extended family, and next-door neighbors would all learn I'm a pothead!

I had sent Chapter 1 of my book to the opinion pages of the *New York Times*, but because of the volume of submissions, I didn't think it would be chosen. When it was accepted, I didn't think it would be published. Even as I read through the copy edits, I expected some world event to take priority. But at 7 am on Thursday March 19, 2015, "How I Buy Weed" went live in the Opinionator, and on March 22 it appeared in print in the *Sunday Review*.

From then on, I knew, marijuana might be the first thing anyone thought about me—and I didn't mind. I was proud to be an advocate. My habit wouldn't cost me my job, because I wouldn't fire myself, and at the time I lived in a state where the penalty for possessing an ounce or less was a $100 ticket. (Now recreational use is legal in New York State.)

I mention these things because people have said I was brave. I was not.

I did lose my biggest writing client, a pharmaceutical company, but that was to be expected. Not only are they a conservative group, but cannabis is an affront to their business model.

And what did the neighbors think?

One ran over to say, "I never knew you smoked! Why didn't you ever offer me any?" Another told me smoking pot is the one thing that helps her seventeen-year-old bipolar son. A third asked if I would address her book club.

I think there are a lot of secret smokers out there: happy and successful individuals who happen to smoke weed. They should leave the closet, if they can.

When gays came out, laws changed. At the federal level, marijuana laws aren't changing fast enough. Cannabis is still a Schedule 1 drug, which means it's classified like heroin or methaqualone, as a drug with no currently accepted medical use (despite being used for healing for five thousand years) and a high potential for misuse (despite its impeccable safety record: no one has ever died from smoking pot).

So consider "voting green" (that is, voting for candidates who are committed to legalization)—and see if you can come out green yourself.

2
Mommy and Me and Marijuana

My husband was very supportive. My three grown sons felt some mixture of pride, amusement, and embarrassment about my marijuana book, which had been featured in popular publications and websites. My friends were happy for me in my new role as a marijuana advocate.

But my aged mom did not approve.

You would think at that point it wouldn't matter. After all, I was collecting Social Security myself. Barcroft TV, a UK outfit, made a short documentary about me with the demeaning title, "Potty Pensioner Puffs A Joint A Day For Fifty Years."

Still, I wanted my nonagenarian mother to encourage my candor about cannabis.

After all, we had so much in common. She was always a free-spirit, a bohemian, a woman of the senses. Like me, she was a writer, and her subject of choice was the French author Colette, who celebrates touch, taste, smell—senses marijuana enhances. Like me, my mother was passionate about various causes, such as preserving old houses and curbing gardening noise. Why didn't she have more sympathy for cannabis legalization?

Her dry assessment of my book? "Well, I liked it more than I intended."

In all fairness, she had given pot a try. I got her high once or twice, with great difficulty, for she had trouble with the smoking process. She coughed a lot and seemed to believe that tilting her head back, rather than inhaling, would bring smoke into her lungs. Once high, she was merry and talkative—pretty much the same way she was usually merry and talkative.

A few years ago, while traveling together in Hawaii, my oldest son gave my mother a marijuana cookie. Then they drove around the island in their rented convertible. From my son's account:

As we're driving the sun is setting, and I've got Thievery Corporation on the stereo. My very cool grandmother, who has never liked ANY electronic music, turns to me and goes: "This music is soooooooo good!" I cracked up. Pretty soon she's telling me "I get it, I really get it! I know why everyone likes marijuana!" It wasn't long before she was asking for some water, and then more or less fell asleep.

But while my mother enjoyed these experiences, she didn't approve of regular use. She wasn't sure marijuana should be legalized, because she didn't like the idea of children getting stoned. I exploded, "Nobody likes that idea! But there will be strict age limits."

She herself was a "high on life" kind of person, although she was too sophisticated to put it like that. She didn't have the need to enhance, or escape from, reality. She got no particular pleasure from alcohol, either: what was the point when life was so exciting and hilarious just as it was?

"Not everyone has that outlook, Mom. Not everyone is as lucky as you."

A week after that conversation, my mom read an article in the *New Yorker* which said that Blacks and whites use weed at comparable rates but in state prisons, there are significant racial disparities in "low level drug offenders—possession of marijuana or drug paraphernalia." In New York state, a Black was 4.5 times as likely as a white to be arrested for weed.

And for a few days my mother's attitude changed. I even got an email saying she was proud of me for fighting injustice. Then Pope Francis became her new crush, because of his environmental encyclical, and my mother slipped back into her usual disdain for marijuana.

Soon after *Just Say Yes* was published, I gave a reading at Canio's Bookstore in Sag Harbor, where she lived. Well into the Q & A, she stood up, clambered onto the stage, and pronounced, "I just want you all to know that I do not endorse my daughter's ideas!"

How I wish she could totter onto a stage and denounce this book now, in her charming and vivacious way! She died in 2022, at age 98, looking out at blue water—the same view I face now as I write this.

3
Cannabis Thought Experiment

America's drinking culture is so ubiquitous we scarcely even notice it. Wine, beer, spirits, cocktails: they're all around us all the time, with their promise of camaraderie, fun, and romance. So alluring! I've always regretted that my physiology doesn't allow me to drink. Alas, alcohol usually makes me faint or nauseous long before it makes me happy.

Luckily, there's a benign alternative, a high that my body (and soul!) embraces. Cannabis is my intoxicant of choice, and although the legalization movement is spreading, most people I know don't smoke openly. So I generally feel bereft when people gather to have fun. They're always urging me to have some wine or a drink, and I usually end up holding a glass of something—the same something all evening long.

To illustrate how alcohol pervades our culture, please join me in a thought experiment. Let's pretend that the history of marijuana and alcohol were reversed, so that marijuana was widely embraced but recreational alcohol (as opposed to medicinal or rubbing alcohol) was banned in many states. In most of America, owning or selling recreational alcohol could put you behind bars, while using marijuana was not only the norm but was culturally celebrated.

If that were the case, your vacation in St. John, a U.S. Virgin Island, might look something like the following. Note: you are not going there specifically to smoke a lot of pot. Marijuana just happens to be everywhere, as it is at most vacation destinations.

After you get off the plane in St. Thomas, you notice that in one corner of the airport by the baggage claim there's a table upon which is displayed a variety of cannabis products: buds, candies, tinctures. All are for sale. A pretty woman is handing out free joints made with the local marijuana. "Welcome to the Virgin Islands," she says. Some tourists light up there and then, while others slip their welcome joints into their pockets. On the ferry to St. John, the first mate comes around to offer passengers marijuana cigarettes and spliffs (which combine pot and tobacco). These, too, are complimentary.

You arrive at the resort, and when you get to your room, you see a bowl of fruit, as well as a small tray holding a grinder, rolling papers, and a lighter. A note reads, "Enjoy Your Stay! The Management." The refrigerator holds soft drinks, peanuts, and various cannabis strains and snacks. You'll be charged handsomely if you avail yourself of these offerings, but hey, you're on vacation!

By now, you're really getting into the island mood or mode, and when go down to the restaurant for dinner, the menu offers yet more cannabis: a chicken marijuana/mole; a pineapple/cannabis upside-down cake. You've already smoked so much free stuff it seems excessive to get it in your food, so you order the fish with mango chutney.

Various joints are offered before, during, and after your meal. These vary by THC and CBD content and by their terpenes. Some strains taste lemony; others taste almost sweet. You are not a cannabis connoisseur yourself, and you're bemused by this emphasis on taste. After all, it's the effect, not the taste, that you're after.

The next day, you head down to the beach. Just as the resort website has depicted, there are two beach chairs set in shallow waters, romantically touching, facing out to sea, complete with hot young couple sharing a bong. Other people float by on rafts, conspicuously puffing from long pipes. All enjoy displaying their consumption.

You decide to go for a sail on a sunset cruise, and immediately upon setting foot on deck, every passenger crowds around the bar, ignoring the plates of shrimp, the bowls of guacamole, the platters of cheese, and the trays of cookies. No, they need to smoke something at once, and they shout their orders to the bud-tender, who supplies them with cannabis products. Fifteen minutes later, the people are mellow and calm. They're delighting in the water, the clouds, the passing islands, the wind—and suddenly, with little shrieks of delight, the food. Later, upon landing at the dock, many passengers go to the upstairs restaurant with its wonderful views. Happy with themselves, each other and the world, they smoke yet again.

At this point, you may be thinking, Who are these crazy potheads—and how much cannabis can they consume in one day? But go back to the early part of this piece, where you land in St. Thomas, and substitute "rum punch" or "wine" or "cocktails" every time you read "cannabis" or "marijuana," and see how normal it all seems. After all, almost every hotel room in America comes equipped with wineglasses, an ice bucket, and a corkscrew.

Let's resume the thought experiment. Coming home from your toking vacation in St. John, you go through security in St. Thomas without a problem, but ahead of you there is some sort of trouble. The local police are converging upon a young college couple. A scan of his backpack has revealed a steel flask; upon examination, it is found to be filled with the illicit island whiskey. The girl has started crying, and no wonder. It's likely they'll both be arrested, and they may be imprisoned for years.

4
A Stoner in St. John

It's the second year I'm here with my mom at Caneel Bay Resort, a one-time Rockefeller establishment in St. John, US Virgin Islands. We are both senior citizens. My small claim to fame is a single publicly-admitted metric: I've smoked pot almost every day for 50 years. I feel it has only enhanced my life. The first edition of my book *Just Say Yes* attests to a happy relationship with cannabis from the first, when I was a college freshman. My aim in coming out has always been to legitimatize pot.

So I decide that this year on vacation, I will be open about my marijuana use. Last year, I was very impressed by the honesty in St. John. I paid for a $10 taxi to Cruz Bay, got out and entered a restaurant. I was surprised a few minutes later, when the taxi driver appeared. He had parked his car and searched me out to hand me what I'd mistakenly given him: a hundred-dollar bill! Similarly, when I lost my watch near the dive shop, a week later, a guide got in touch with me through my website and mailed it back.

This year, I walk the half-mile path to the dive shop to thank him in person. He isn't there, but I wait to speak to another guide. Suddenly, he wrinkles his nose and goes out to the beach to tell a tourist to put out his cigarette. "I hate that smell," he says. Then he asks me, "Do you smoke?"

I say, "Only weed."

A huge smile blooms on his face. Up goes his hand for a happy high-five. Our commonality becomes a bridge that spans our forty-year age difference. I inquire about the local stuff, and he says he can get me an eighth for forty. I write my cell number down for him. I've made a connection and now I don't have to be so frugal with what I've brought down, which is really not enough.

That night, I board the resort shuttle bus to get to my room. I'm the only passenger, and the driver says, "You are gorgeous! Can I get your autograph?"

Friends, when you are collecting social security, these moments are not scorned but cherished. "You are sweet," I say. And since I am very buzzed from a single rum drink, I tell him about my book and its title. When he hears "A marijuana memoir," his whole face lights up. He says, "Guess what? I drive around here stoned all day."

Who can blame him? He's working in paradise. And driving a shuttle bus at 15 miles an hour on roads through these two hundred pristine acres isn't very demanding. A slow-moving donkey might be the only obstacle. At the shuttle stop, the driver helps me down from the bus, and I go to my room to give him a copy of my book, which I sign with a flourish. I decide to keep on being open and see where it gets me.

One thing it does not get me is more pot! The guy from the dive shop never calls me, and having smoked with abandon when I thought I'd get more, I now have only two joints for four days. As I love to get stoned and snorkel, which one can do from the beach here, I'm on extreme rations. For this reason, I'm not stoned when our next-door neighbor, June, comes over. She's heard the Women's March playing on my iPad on my patio, and she wants to watch with me. She's about my age, earnest, plain, a New England type. A Quaker, I call her to myself, although I have no idea of her faith. We listen to some speeches, and after an hour, she goes back to her room.

The next day, we run into June and her husband at afternoon tea, which is held on a terrace overlooking the sea. We sit with them, and she asks what I write. My mother gets a worried look on her face. She was quite a bohemian in her day, so she's never been shocked at my marijuana use. Still, she's socially uncomfortable with my present life as an advocate. I want to please her (yes, even at my age!), but I also don't want to hide an important part of my recent life.

"I write novels," I say, "but no one's ever paid any attention to my books until the latest one, *Just Say Yes: A Marijuana Memoir*."

I examine June's face. There's no trace of disapproval there, and I see my mother start to relax. Our new friend glances at her husband and says, "We used to use it when we went hiking, didn't we, dear?" She is very matter of fact. "Weed is so much lighter than wine."

I have to laugh. There are many reasons for smoking instead of drinking: a mellower high, more creativity, no blackouts, no hangover, no aggression. In all this time, however, I have never considered something as practical as marijuana's portability!

On our last morning, the shuttle bus takes us down to the buffet breakfast. There are two couples on the bus, and my mom and me. The couples leave first. My mom and I are slower. We are in pants because soon we will travel. We descend the stairs cautiously. Then I see the driver, the one from the other night. He gives me a wink. Then he reaches under the dashboard to wave my book at me.

5
The Intermission Joint

Of course, I would have to get high before the John Lennon tribute concert at Symphony Space a few years ago. That was never at issue. Music and marijuana are a sacred duo, with the latter always enhancing the former. But how would I stay high? I decided I would just slip out at intermission, find a doorway on a side street, and light up.

I know, I know, this may seem reckless and juvenile, especially at my great age. Still, I've been smoking for decades on the streets of New York City, and I've never been caught or even approached. If a cop ever got near, I would just drop the joint and grind it out with my shoe. There would be nothing else on me because I never carry more than a single joint.

Smoking pot seemed especially appropriate before—and during—a tribute to John Lennon, who loved cannabis and greatly influenced the hippie culture. I imbibed in the car as we came down from Westchester. My triathlete husband drove; he smokes only rarely and just for medical reasons: he says it prevents his legs from cramping after long runs.

Going to Symphony Space, I had my hand out the window because the smell of pot lingers for weeks in a car's upholstery.

We parked on Riverside Drive and walked to the theater. As expected, the people streaming into the venue were mainly in late middle age or older. After all, we were the ones John Lennon most affected; had he lived, he would have been seventy-five that night. Most of the concert performers, although younger, were also past first youth and had been touring for years. We knew them from when we were "young," in our forties, and from festivals like Clearwater.

Even from the balcony, we had a great view of the stage, and the performers were terrific. Martin Sexton, Lucy Kaplansky, Willie Nile, Joan Osborn: what superb voices and songs! There was also a tall, handsome musician I'd never heard of. He really cooked, but I forgot his name as soon as it was announced. Some names are like that: they just disappear.

Soon it was intermission and time for my maintenance smoke. "See you soon," I told my husband as I left the theater.

I turned the corner and found myself on 95th Street. It wasn't long before I was in a good doorway. It was mild for December, so I wasn't wearing gloves. Out came the lighter, out came the joint, and soon I was blazing. All was fine and getting finer when some guy suddenly approached and said, "Hey, can I have some of that?"

"Uh . . . no!"

"Oh, come on."

"But I don't know you!"

"Weren't you just at that concert?"

I nodded.

"Well, you just saw me play!" It was the tall, handsome musician. And he told me his name, which was so bland (two first names, like Paul George) I promptly forgot it again. I passed him the joint. Oh, this was cozy, toking up with a cute performer while my husband awaited me inside! Then the man burst my bubble by saying, "Can I call my girlfriend to come over?"

"There's not enough!" I cried. "I have only this one joint!"

It was mostly gone by now, so he didn't persist, just took a long toke. Then he said, "We just came in from Canada, and we don't know people in New York."

"I wish I had more weed for you, but I'm always very cautious on the streets."

"Yeah, like now," he teased. He passed me the roach, which was small and dead. I put it in my pocket.

"Hey, thanks," he said. "Nice smoke!"

I returned to the theater and my seat. "How did it go?" asked my husband.

"It was fabulous! A lifetime fantasy of mine just came true, at the age of sixty-nine! I smoked a joint with one of the performers!"

"Wow," he said. "Which one?"

Uh, hmm, um, blush. Memory loss? Inattention? Cannabis fog? I didn't want to admit to any of these, and I didn't want to say "I forget."

I found the name in the program and was armed with an answer when he asked again.

6
How I (Used to) Buy Weed

Ephraim's place is a few blocks above 96th Street on the East Side, where the neighborhood is rundown but not dangerous. There's no intercom in the building, so to open the downstairs door, you have to have your own key. Ephraim doesn't take phone calls on either landline or cell. Ephraim doesn't use the internet. Ephraim stays under the radar.

Ephraim is 63, with curly gray hair that he wears in a thick ponytail. He has regular hours and regular customers. He accepts new clients reluctantly, and only if they are the good friends or adult children of his existing customers. Ephraim is honest, good-natured and very, very careful.

Ephraim is an important person in my life. He is my dealer. Ephraim has been dealing grass, and only grass, from this one location for 35 years. He has been my personal supplier for almost that long. I go down to his place every couple of months, but some of his customers visit twice a week. These must be lower-level dealers. My standard purchase of an ounce or two is dwarfed by what the others are buying.

Ephraim provides a valued service to us all.

To keep squeaky clean, Ephraim has a really boring day job so he can show taxable income to the IRS. He's had this job for decades, although he must clear a quarter of a million a year dealing grass. I arrive at this figure based on estimated client volume, average buy and a 40 percent mark-up.

Anyway, Ephraim is certainly doing well. And doing good.

It's easy to park in Ephraim's neighborhood, so I always drive down from Westchester, with a novel on audio. On this Monday night, I park right across the street from his building. His downstairs door is painted a bright, acrylic yellow. I insert my key and turn the lock. The door opens smartly—upon the dirtiest hallway I have ever seen. The white hexagonal tiles have not been washed in decades. Crumpled wrappers and unidentifiable filth have been ground into the grime. As always, I breathe through my mouth, between my teeth.

The stairway is no better. The brown linoleum is broken and littered with cigarette butts. The walls are covered with graffiti, and there are five flights of stairs. Most of Ephraim's customers are in late middle age, and I wonder how much longer we'll be able to make it up these stairs. I picture us coming up in knee braces, gripping the banisters, panting.

I get to his floor without pausing or gasping, but my heart is definitely going fast, and I rest a moment to catch my breath. Then I push his doorbell.

It's one of those bells that gives no indication about whether or not it works. There's no buzz and there's no light, so sometimes when I don't hear movement inside, I press the bell again, certain that it hasn't worked the first time. This gets Ephraim annoyed, so tonight I just wait. And yes, I do hear noises now: the click of the peephole opening, the clunk of the floor lock-bar being moved. The door opens, and he beckons me in, finger to lips Ephraim insists on silence at his door. He doesn't want his neighbors to be aware of the many visitors he gets Monday to Thursday between eight and ten pm. He calls these his "office hours," and this hovel is his office. He lives elsewhere with his wife and three children, now young adults.

I follow him down the long corridor of this cramped apartment. "How are you?" he asks in his friendly, nasal voice.

We have to go sideways down the hall because of the bicycle. (This will pose a problem when his clients start using walkers.) We get to the studio—and it's 1969, with posters, books and vinyl record albums from that era. Three old hippie-types sprawl on two ancient couches. The small room has been partitioned into two areas. There's the outer area, where customers wait for Ephraim's attentions. And through an open doorway there's the inner area, where Ephraim sits at a desk, underneath a loft bed, weighing the goods. When you first get in there with him, it's like entering a cave.

I nod to the others, a weathered lot, all of us. I've seen one of the guys here before—Hank, I think—and the others look vaguely familiar. Friends of Ephraim. We should have a club. We should throw him a party.

Ephraim says, "Come on in, Hank," and they go into the inner area. The rest of us make small talk. There's always a festive atmosphere at Ephraim's. Martha, with the long gray hair, is an artist who lives in Williamsburg. Richard, who is bald, teaches music at a junior high school. I inject a note of politics into the chitchat, certain that they share my leftie views, which they do.

Hank is in the inner area with Ephraim for ten minutes. He gets four ounces of Mex and two ounces of sensi. He emerges into the outer area and puts his purchases into a backpack. He shakes hands with Richard, nods to Martha and me and says to Ephraim, "See you Thursday."

A dealer for sure.

It's Richard's turn. Richard wants half a pound of hydro-ponic, which Ephraim gets by coming into the outer area and opening a small refrigerator with no shelves in its interior. At any time, Ephraim has between ten and twenty pounds of pot from five or six locales, and he keeps it in large plastic bags in a dormitory refrigerator. He takes out one of the bags and closes the refrigerator door. Ephraim reaches into the bag and draws out a branchlet of marijuana. He shows it to Martha. "Pretty," she croons. The buds are red and sticky with resin. Ephraim goes back into the inner area with Richard.

Martha talks about her paintings and gives me a postcard for the opening of her next show. Then she goes in to see Ephraim.

Finally, it's my turn. By now, two new customers, guys, have joined us, heralded each time by the piercing buzzer. I can see why it irritates Ephraim when people push it twice. One of the new guys is very young, scarcely forty. I go into the inner area.

Ephraim looks up at me from under the low ceiling of the loft bed, like a friendly, bright animal. "What's it going to be? The usual?"

"Maybe this time I'll buy something exotic."

"Don't bother," he says, as always.

We have had this discussion many times. He maintains that his customers who roll joints—as opposed to those who use a pipe—should just buy the Mexican. Why pay two or three times as much when so much of it will be wasted, going up in smoke? The cheap stuff costs $140 an ounce, and that's what he always insists that I buy.

It's an unusual merchant who steers you away from his more expensive lines.

"I need two ounces this time. I'm buying some for this couple in their eighties."

"Very cool," says Ephraim.

He weighs my economy pot on a metal balance scale. He hasn't gone digital yet. He asks about my work and my children. "My youngest son wants to meet you," I say. "He can't believe your prices."

It's been many years since Ephraim has raised his prices, reputedly the lowest in the city. "Your son is how old?" asks Ephraim.

"Twenty-nine."

"Sure. Bring him down with you next time." Ephraim insists on a personal introduction. Then he asks, "Does he still ski?"

Ephraim is very good about remembering that sort of

thing. Then again, he's had essentially the same client base for decades.

"Oh yes," I tell him. "Jerome's a treat to watch. Like a velvet ribbon unspooling."

"How about you?" asks Ephraim.

"I ski mainly cross-country now."

Ephraim gives me my dope in a plastic baggie, and I hand over the bills, crisp twenties fresh from the bank. I put the baggie in my handbag.

He stands up and takes out a fat roll of cash from his shirt pocket. He tucks my bills under the rubber band with the others and puts his roll back in his pocket. He makes a tiny jotting into a small notebook, and he walks me to the outer room. I say goodbye to the other dopers and edge down the hallway with my host, past the bicycle.

Ephraim opens the door and we part cordially and silently.

On my way down the filthy stairs, I put my wallet into my coat pocket. When I get to the car, I put my handbag in the trunk. I take this precaution in case a traffic cop asks to see my license and registration. This way, I'll just reach into my pocket for my wallet instead of into a handbag fragrant with weed.

In my own way, I'm pretty careful myself. I would never go to Ephraim's with a broken taillight or an outdated inspection ticket, for never am I so vulnerable to the law as when I am returning home with a fresh stash.

I turn on the engine, activating narration. I scarcely go anywhere without fiction.

Half an hour later, I'm in my driveway in Westchester. I

open the trunk and reach for my handbag. I've made another drug run to the city. I've scored again. I'm stoked and psyched. I'm set for another eight weeks.

7
An Ounce for the
Octogenarians

A few days before I visit Ephraim, my aunt, who is 92 and lives near me, asks if she can come over. She wants to talk about something confidential. She still drives, and like several of her friends, she is active, able and productive. As I wait for her, I wonder what's on her mind. Perhaps it has something to do with her sister, my mother, who lives on her own in Sag Harbor. Or perhaps my aunt, who has written several mystery novels, wants some editing advice.

It's Saturday. My husband helps my aunt up the front steps and goes off for a run. My aunt and I sit down in the living room. "I'm really here on behalf of my friend Lois," she tells me. "She has rheumatoid arthritis, and she's in terrible pain. She's been in pain for years."

I see where this conversation is headed.

My aunt continues. "Her doctor says many people like her get relief from medical marijuana, but . . ." She gives me a helpless look.

"But she doesn't know how to get any," I conclude.

She nods. "I thought perhaps you might be able to help."

Everyone in my family knows I smoke pot (although probably not how much). I say, "Sure, glad to help." It's almost time for me to visit Ephraim anyway, so I'll just buy a little more.

"Lois will be so grateful. She was very surprised to hear the doctor recommend it, and she didn't know who to ask."

"It's ridiculous that pot should be illegal," I say, "when it brings so many people such relief. And it's not like you can overdose on it. Or even get a hangover."

"It may not work, you know."

"Perhaps not, but she should give it a try. Especially if her doctor recommended it. Tell her to call me, and we'll work out the details."

My aunt leaves, and Lois calls within the hour. She has a pleasant, youthful voice. I suggest that she drop off the money the next day, as Ephraim's is strictly a cash business. She seems pleased with the arrangement.

On Sunday, Lois and her husband, George, a psychotherapist, come up the front steps. They're a bit younger than my aunt—sprightly, in their early eighties—so they don't need my husband's assistance. He lets them in and calls me to come down from the study. He shouts upstairs to me, "I'll be back in an hour."

I come downstairs to meet Lois and George. They are a very natty, well-groomed couple, casually dressed in pressed cotton clothes. Her blond hair is nicely coiffed, and she wears red lipstick; his hat is set at a jaunty angle. My aunt has told me he still has a private practice. It's a warm Sunday, so I take them to the back porch where, rather than the usual white wicker with blue chintz, I've tried for a Moroccan look. We sink into the porch chairs, which are a deep brown with red cushions. In the middle of the chairs is a round, tiled coffee table with an intricate Islamic pattern at which I can stare for minutes on end, especially when I'm high, enjoying figure/ground reversals.

Lois says, brightly, warmly, to break the ice, "I just saw your son going off for his run."

I hear myself actually make the sound, "Grrrrr!" Then I say, "That's my husband!"

Lois looks embarrassed.

I say, "That's okay." It's annoying, but understandable. Mark does have a baby face, and he is 16 years younger, a difference I often ignore because he's so caring—even fatherly—with me.

Changing the subject hastily, George says, "Here's the money." He hands me an envelope with bills inside.

"Great. I'll be visiting my dealer sometime next week."

"What form does it come in?" he asks.

"Just a minute, I'll show you." I go to the freezer and take out my remaining quarter ounce, which is in a baggie surrounded by a brown paper lunch bag surrounded by a Tupperware container. I bring out the container and reveal the small, dense mass of dried yet dampish leaves.

"How do you smoke that?" asks George.

"First, have you smoked cigarettes before?"

"We smoked *pot* before," says George, to my surprise. "A long time ago."

"It used to be very relaxing," says Lois. "We liked it."

"I don't know why we stopped," said George. "But we know it agrees with Lois. And if it will take away some of her pain…"

"It's certainly worth trying," I say. I'm relieved that they have some familiarity with pot's effects; it makes me less responsible in case anything goes wrong. But what could go wrong? She'd fall asleep?

"I'll be right back." I get my marijuana accoutrements and return to the vibrant octogenarians on my back porch. I tell them, "You can smoke it in a pipe or as a cigarette. If you smoke a pipe, you just break off a piece of this compacted mass and put it in the bowl." I show them the small glass pipe my middle son, Simon, bought me, and stuff a little grass into it. "Personally, I like joints. You don't have to keep fussing around with the lighting, and you're always smoking clean grass, not char."

"We like joints, too, don't we dear?"

Lois nods. George says, "That's what we used to smoke. So what do we do, grind it up?"

"I rub it through a strainer, like this." I put a little pot into a metal strainer, which I place over a stainless steel mixing bowl. I start pushing it back and forth, until I have a small pile of cleaned pot underneath the strainer. I put this into an old plastic film can. They watch with interest as I take out a packet of cigarette papers.

"Where would I get papers?" asks George. I notice he's asking all the questions.

"Many places. Most gas stations have them. Get size 1¼ or 1½." I extract a paper from my pack of 1¼ e-z widers. I say, "Glue side up," and tap out a line of marijuana from the film can into the crease. "Go back and forth a bit to firm it up"—I show them how with my thumbs—"then roll it for real and seal it up." I lick the glue and press the joint closed. "Voila!"

Then George asks a curious question. I smile and say, "Absolutely." I hand him the joint. "You might as well have this."

He thanks me profusely and slips it into his shirt pocket. Lois thanks me, too.

I joke, "I hope you can wait until you get home before smoking it."

"We can do that," says George.

My aunt calls me later that night. She asks, "Did everything go well with George and Lois?"

"Oh, yes. They're such a nice couple. I gave them a little class in cleaning and rolling marijuana. Then I gave them a joint."

"That was very sweet of you, dear."

"You know, auntie, I don't think they want it for strictly medicinal reasons."

She says, "What do you mean?"

"I think they want to use it 'recreationally.' They just want to get high again. Especially George."

"You *would* think that," my aunt chides. "But that's non-sense! Whatever gave you that idea?"

"Because when I showed George how to roll a joint, he asked me anxiously, 'Will one joint be enough for two people?'"

8
Celebration

I wish drink did the trick, I really do. People in bars look like they're having a wonderful time, and people at parties laugh a lot more after drinking. But, like several other women in my family, I don't tolerate alcohol well, so marijuana is my inebriant of choice.

It should be no more significant than that. Instead, the millions of people who smoke pot routinely must be furtive about their habit because in most parts of the world, and in most of the United States, there are legal and financial penalties for smoking pot. In 2014, three-quarters of a million people in the USA were behind bars for marijuana offenses. Costs vary from state to state, but on average it cost taxpayers about $47,000 per prisoner. We could have saved $33 billion a year simply by pardoning all the inmates who were in prison because of marijuana. This wouldn't have saved only money: it would have saved lives. It is profoundly unjust that so many (principally minority youth) were in jail because they owned or trafficked in an herb that gives pleasure to so many.

There are also social penalties, so smokers tend to be quiet about their habit. Along with the secrecy comes a certain shame, at least for people past a certain age, at least about habitual smoking.

I write this account to counteract that shame. I think it's time for a positive narrative about long-term cannabis use. As someone who's indulged for some fifty years, I'm glad to publish this memoir under my own name. It's high time marijuana habitués came out of the closet—hat's off to Bill Maher! Pot use should be normalized. Weed is not something exotic, and smoking pot doesn't mean you're peculiar. When gays started coming out, the laws changed. I believe that people who get high should be more open about it, within their risk tolerance. That's what fuels this memoir.

Additionally, I'm drawn to the literary challenge of organizing the events of my life as they relate to marijuana—and (sadly? gladly?) it isn't much of a stretch. Weed is the spine of this memoir as drink is the center of so many others, such as Caroline Knapp's *Drinking: A Love Story,* Pete Hamill's *A Drinking Life,* Barbara Holland's *The Joy of Drinking* and Mary Karr's *Lit.*

Reverse chronology seems the only way I can write this. For one thing, I wouldn't want the reader to expect the usual narrative arc. I do not end up in prison. My life isn't ruined. I do not regret my years of lighting up. On the contrary.

Let me center this memoir by celebrating its effects on me. These have been much the same for decades. Of course there are downsides to smoking, which another chapter will address.

For now, I celebrate without restraint the sacred herb, the holy weed, the blessed hemp.

How do I use it? Let me count the ways.

For inspiration and writing. After half a joint (of that lousy Mexican stuff I always buy), I feel a tingling in my elbows and a warm general confidence. Happiness suffuses my brain, and I become more playful and inventive. It's the perfect time to plan a project, because ideas come more quickly. It's also a good time to actually write, because I usually feel so good I don't notice the demons of doubt. Being high eases me into writing; after a while, I'm no longer stoned, but the writing momentum continues. I'm in flow.

I also like being high for the final read-through, of either my own fiction or pieces I edit or write for others. I honestly feel I owe it to my clients to do the final reading after smoking, for then I often see subtle infelicities of meaning or rhythm that I've missed before, and I correct them on the spot. I do not usually check again when I'm straight, as I'm confident about my fine-tuning decisions while stoned. I give my clients a perk they know nothing about: a high level of attention.

Of course, I don't smoke just for writing and editing. Basically, weed is a general pleasure drug for me, a mild, reliable way to get happy. Most things I enjoy I enjoy even more when I'm high, especially if they don't require energy. So relaxing outdoors is especially good for me after smoking. I like being baked while I lie on the beach, being stoned when I stroll in a drizzle and being high when I walk in the sun upon new fallen snow.

Kayaking at sunset is reliably wonderful, but marijuana brings it to aesthetic and spiritual bliss. I paddle mainly in the calm harbor near my house, slowly, at the end of the day. Sometimes other boaters ask, "Are you as happy as you look?" and I always nod yes. Paddling like this is more meditation than sport. When people ask if kayaking is difficult, I sometimes say, "The hardest part is lighting the joint in the wind."

I wonder if the harbor police have ever seen me hunched and struggling. Probably: when I wave my paddle at them, they do not wave in return.

I get high for many of the good things in life—and none of the bad. Pot is an intensifier: as it augments the good, so it deepens the ugly, the bleak, the depressing. For me, it makes bad things worse. So the contention that getting high is an escape from one's problems is irrelevant to me. I smoke to augment pleasure, not to dull pain.

Snorkeling in a coral reef is one of the best things of all to do stoned. There you are, drifting along in warm water, the sun on your back, your face in what seems like a vast aquarium, while fish of all sizes and colors swim just beneath you, sometimes by the hundreds. And all you need to do is move a lazy flipper now and then and watch the show unfold. It is all beauty and comfort, no threat, and being stoned makes it even more ecstatic.

But I would never scuba dive stoned: too much anxiety about breathing!

Some people like to run or bike when they're stoned, but I don't like to be physically active. Smoking makes me languorous and passive. That's probably why I like weed so much. I tend to be a speedy person, with, I was once told, exophthalmic eyes. I'm very active, sometimes driven; pot calms and cocoons me. "Life is always a tightrope or a featherbed," wrote Edith Wharton. "Give me the tightrope." But I like pot because it brings me down from the wire and onto a pillow. It's great as a calming agent after an ordeal, such as a rough drive home, and it's a fine way to start the weekend.

It opens the senses. There are three things people traditionally enjoy after smoking weed: listening to music, eating and making love. Perhaps pot lets one focus more fully on a single sense: when I'm high I feel I listen more attentively, more fully, with music pouring into my very soul. I love to hear Bach in a church, for the ambience and the acoustics, so just before the concert I'll be sneaking around the perimeter of the church parking lot, or ducking between rows of cars, surreptitiously toking up before entering the space. I wonder if anybody smells marijuana on my hair or coat. I wonder if others are high, too. When I'm stoned, I like following instruments individually, first one, then another. Am I really hearing better? Who knows? I do feel I'm more in the moment.

Many philosophers feel that living in the moment is the key to happiness. Perhaps that's why I love to smoke: it keeps me alive in the present.

When I'm high, my taste buds become exquisitely sensitive, and I appreciate food even more than usual. I am more attuned to its texture and flavor: I can taste the carrot in the sauce like following the bass in a song. I consider it a disservice to a fine restaurant to dine there without being high. Even on an ordinary weeknight, I usually smoke pot before dinner, the way others have a cocktail on returning home from work. Pot makes food tastes better: it's my reward to myself as the cook.

Having sex is the third sacred thing to do stoned, at least for many. Skin becomes more sensitive, kissing more complex, anything oral more interesting and compelling. And the feet! When I'm high and Mark squeezes my arches and pulls my toes, I'm in heaven. But while pot is great for making out and fooling around, for me it's not good for making love. Marijuana dries the eyes, the mouth and the vagina. Then there's that pot-induced self-consciousness: the constant mental commentary, the racing mind. For one reason or another, I'm less orgasmic when I'm high.

But I like the spontaneity, even the goofiness, pot fosters between people. So I like to get high with friends (those few who still smoke) because our conversations will be more whimsical and will seem more hilarious. Are they "in fact" more hilarious? Probably not, but so what? If the conversation leads to laughter and joy, does it really matter that someone who hasn't smoked might not find it as funny as we do? It's not as if anything depends upon the actual wittiness of our discourse. We're not creating art—or a script for *Saturday Night Live*. We're just hanging out, having fun.

For that matter, is there a difference between seeming to be happy and actually being happy? Or: if you think you're happy—aren't you?

9
Downside

Even a pothead like me knows that marijuana isn't wholly salubrious. My habit has many drawbacks. These, and economics, check any impulse I might have to smoke even more than I do.

Pot makes me sleepy and lethargic, especially two hours after smoking. The fatigue aspect means it's not a good idea for me to smoke before mid-afternoon. If I smoke before dinner as well, I might start yawning by ten. Weed is not good if I want to party hearty or simply stay awake until eleven. (Pot-smokers rarely suffer from insomnia.) Furthermore, marijuana dulls the dreams. My friend Sophia claims that whenever she goes on a marijuana fast and stops smoking pot, her dreams are more colorful, more complex, more fully fleshed. Best of all, she remembers them. She loves these dreams and misses them most of the year—because, all things considered, like most of us heads, she'd rather get high.

Pot also takes its toll upon one's personal charms. It makes the eyes red, and it may cause wrinkles. I try to smoke with a loose mouth, without pursing my lips, but fine lines are starting to appear anyway. And grass is bad for the breath. Most dopers carry mints to avoid the dreaded dragon breath.

Marijuana famously makes one hungry and makes great food taste even better. This is advantageous if one is too thin or in chemotherapy, but for the rest of us…not so much.

Then there's the memory issue. It's pretty clear from both scientific studies and personal experience that pot impairs short-term memory and learning. Pot makes it harder to retain information or ideas: it's counterproductive to go to class stoned. If I get high before seeing a film, in a couple of weeks, I might not remember anything about it—even that I've seen it. If you get high a lot, those are hours that leave little residue. I worry a lot about this. Isn't memory a sign of intelligence— and what if frequent marijuana use affects long-term memory, too?

Certainly, my memory is worse than it used to be—but most of my contemporaries complain about memory deficits. The average person of 60 remembers only 20 percent as well as the average person of 20. My friends who complain most about losing their memory are only occasional smokers (if that), so I attribute my own memory lapses to age rather than addiction. Nora Ephron was about my age when she wrote her book *I Remember Nothing*, and as far as I know, she was not a marijuana devotee. Still, it's entirely possible that I'd remember a lot more if I smoked a lot less.

At the PEN World Voices Festival, I listen to Lewis Lapham, longtime editor of *Harper's*, participate in the "Obsessions" series. His own obsession is smoking cigarettes. He started at 17 because it was cool and there was the connotation of fellow-feeling: you offered one to strangers, to women, and it was "a delight." He believes that nicotine makes the mind sharper, and he regards the antismoking movement as oppressing the poor. He notes that Hitler tried to restrict smokers. Lapham resents the efforts of the state to tell smokers what to do. "The freedoms in this country have been diminished in my lifetime," he says. "Most people are photographed some forty-five times a day." Lapham, in his late seventies, doesn't believe that cigarette smoking is harmful to all people, only those with certain genes. His own doctor says it isn't hurting him. Nonetheless, I can't help noticing that Lapham has a chronic cough. I feel he's a charming gentleman—in heavy denial.

Am I in denial myself?

If I continue smoking while acknowledging that pot saps my energy and makes my eyes red and my breath bad and impairs short term memory—if I go on toking up every day despite these things, perhaps it's not a habit but an addiction. Certainly, I feel a vague unease if 24 hours pass and I haven't gotten high, and I always replenish my supply before running out. Granted, I'm dependent on pot, but am I an addict? Curious, I ponder the questions from the page from a government website: www.easyread.drugabuse.gov

Do You or a Loved One
Have a Drug Abuse Problem?

Here are some questions to ask yourself or someone you know. If the answer to some or all of these questions is yes, you might have an addiction.

1. Do you think a lot about drugs?

2. Did you ever try to stop or cut down on your drug use but couldn't?

3. Have you ever thought you couldn't fit in or have a good time without drugs?

4. Do you ever use drugs because you are upset or angry at other people?

5. Have you ever used a drug without knowing what it was or what it would do to you?

6. Have you ever taken one drug to get over the effects of another?

7. Have you ever made mistakes at a job or at school because you were using drugs?

8. Does the thought of running out of drugs really scare you?

9. Have you ever stolen drugs or stolen stuff to pay for drugs?

10. Have you ever been arrested or in the hospital because of your drug use?

11. Have you ever overdosed on drugs?

12. Has using drugs hurt your relationships with other people?

Here I am, a senior citizen, saying yes to 1, 2, 3 and 8. I guess that means I am somewhat addicted, which seems about right.

On the list at Narcotics Anonymous there are 29 questions by which you can gauge if you're an addict. I find myself saying yes to eight of them. Here are the new questions to which my answer is yes:

1. Do you ever use alone?

11. Have you ever lied about what or how much you use?

21. Have you ever felt defensive, guilty, or ashamed about your using?

28. Do you continue to use despite negative consequences?

29. Do you think you might have a drug problem?

But here's the thing. Before NA asks you those questions, it declares: "Very simply, an addict is a person whose life is controlled by drugs." And my life certainly isn't. I always have grass on hand and I use it regularly, but my life is not controlled by pot. Similarly, I always have food on hand and I eat three times a day, but my life is not controlled by food.

I once read about a young woman who was offered a wonderful job in Singapore but refused it because the pot penalties there were severe, and she couldn't do without it. Sure, her choice was constrained by her habit: her life *was* to some extent controlled by marijuana. But I can't really see how my life would be any different if I didn't smoke pot.

Okay: I might have more energy. I might also have more insomnia.

Okay: I'd be less paranoid. But is it really paranoia when you're doing something illegal? In New York State, possession of less than an ounce of pot results in just a $100 fine, but the penalty for smoking in public can be three months in jail. What if that person across the alley in the cook's apron is really a cop?

Paranoia tends to stoke an us-and-them mentality. The world becomes divided into pot-smokers and non-pot-smokers. Or into those who'd think less of me if they knew about my habit and those who would not. I know I risk losing some measure of local acceptance by writing my life as a marijuana memoir, but writing against the grain is in my very nature: what's the point of saying what others have said before? Perhaps I'm perverse: even when I write novels and can call on the "fictional alibi," the thought of outraging others is somehow a spur to my process.

But though being an outlaw in my writing seems to satisfy some inner need, risking arrest for possession or smoking in public does not.

But I digress—within a digression.

Have I mentioned that I'm somewhat allergic to pot?

This is a personal downside: I usually start sneezing shortly after smoking—and sometimes when I'm merely cleaning it. Needless to say, this hasn't deterred me from smoking, especially since I like to sneeze. Marijuana is my snuff. Still, perhaps my allergy to cannabis means my eyes get especially red when I smoke weed. I'm always dripping Visine into my eyeballs or wearing sunglasses indoors. If people ask me why my eyes are bloodshot, I say, truthfully, "Allergies."

A final drawback to marijuana is its cost. This is entirely due to it being illegal, for it's easy to grow in most of the country. (Why do you think they call it weed?) Because it's illegal, it's unnaturally expensive. Still, my costs are no more than $100 a month. My husband drinks half a bottle of wine most nights, and like me, he doesn't make expensive choices regarding his preferred inebriant. His dependence costs only a little more than mine. These habits are not financially punishing, and they give us pleasure and peace, so it's likely we'll maintain them. Perhaps we're co-enablers, but we feel we have substance use under control. He's not drinking and I'm not smoking any more than we did five years ago.

We're not cutting back, either. Maybe one day we will.

On October 5, 2024, few months before the 10th Anniversary Edition of this book is published, the *New York Times* runs a long article, "Unexpected Problem in the Rise of Marijuana."

Tens of millions of Americans use cannabis for medical or rec-reational purposes—most of them without problems. But a growing number of people are enduring "serious health con-sequences," including mini-psychotic breaks and uncontrolled vomiting.

I've often observed that cannabis affects everyone differ-ently, with some people getting high at their first puff of a joint and others unaffected by pipeful after pipeful. I never try to persuade a cannabis virgin to smoke pot with me. What if she hates it? Or develops "cannabinoid hyperemesis syndrome"? Far from alleviating nausea, as it usually does, marijuana causes some people to throw up. To alleviate their misery, these people get into hot baths, which somehow help. Now that marijuana is widely legal, hospitals are admitting more and more patients with C.H.S., though nobody I know has ever experienced it.

So, yes. For some, there are downsides to regular (or even one-time) cannabis use.

For me, I exult in the upsides.

10
Are You Getting High Too Often?

Hey, it's possible to overdo any good thing, even getting high! Responsible cannabis use involves setting some boundaries and sometimes saying no. Recreational marijuana should enhance one's life, not muffle or hobble it. All things are not best experienced high!

We all have different lifestyles and tolerance levels, but here are some signs that you just may be using too much. Don't think if you have four yeses you must check into rehab! But if a question resonates with you, you might consider cutting down.

★★★

1. **Is your cannabis consumption interfering with your relationships?** There are various dynamics between people who like pot and people who prefer alcohol—or no intoxicants at all. One of my sons, a therapist, says he prefers to talk to me when I'm straight because he feels I'm more present, so I'm careful not to call him after smoking. Consider whether you'd get along better with someone you love if you didn't consume so much.

2. Is it adversely affecting your productivity?

Is it slowing or dulling your thoughts when you want them to be quick and sharp? You may be using marijuana for inspiration only to find you're routinely falling asleep. For some people, cannabis brings greater clarity and focus; for others (perhaps most of us), it's just the reverse.

3. Does your need to get high stop you from doing things you would otherwise enjoy?

That is, do you have "anti-acrophobia," the fear of not being high? Would you turn down a down a job or vacation if you couldn't use the herb? Do you assess each situation as to whether or not you can get stoned?

4. Is it impacting your memory?

When you're stoned, it's harder to lay down memories. Pot imparts a cozy glow, so it's tempting to reach for the pipe when vegging in front of the TV, but if you light up, you'll probably forget the plot of the movie you're watching (until you fall asleep), and in a few days, you may well forget that you've watched it at all. Your experience has been etched in water.

5. Are you more fatigued than you'd like to be?

Are you yawning at inappropriate times? Are you tired after a day of not much activity? Do you need nine hours' sleep—or more? You might experiment to learn the relationship between your smoking and your energy level.

6. Are you breaking your personal pot rules?

We all have them. Some of us vow that we won't drive or go to work or visit mom when high. Yet suddenly we find we're making exceptions: it's only a mile, it's casual Friday, she'll never even notice. You made those rules for a reason; breaking them means you're losing control of your cannabis use. It's usually better to feel in control.

7. Do you feel guilty about smoking?

Though there's still a certain social stigma to getting high, by now you've probably blown right through it. But perhaps you still beat yourself up about how much you smoke. Perhaps you acknowledge that you should smoke less, but somehow you just can't cut back. This makes you feel guilty, not a good feeling. You have a choice. Get over the guilt or . . . try smoking less. Maybe you don't need that after-dinner joint to relax. Aren't you relaxed enough anyway? Or see what it's like to completely abstain for a while. See what you're like when you're straight.

8. Is your cannabis consumption cutting into your budget?

Whether legal or not, marijuana is expensive. The cheap Mexican at $140 an ounce is a thing of the past, and not everyone can be, or wants to be, a grower. If you get high two or three times a day, you can easily spend $400 a month for the privilege. Is this the best way for you to go through $4,800 a year?

9. Are you not getting as high as you'd like to be?_

Ah, the paradox! More product doesn't lead to more pleasure —only to tolerance. Habituation is the great hedonic demon. One test of good weed is how delightfully different it makes you feel from when you're straight. So how can you really feel high if that's your habitual mode?

Also, smoking more at one time does not necessarily get you higher. The human body is always trying for equilibrium, and if you bombard the cannabis receptors, they're likely to shut down. Once you know this, you have a new fear: are you smoking too *much* to get high? With each batch of weed, what's the optimal amount?

If only to truly enjoy cannabis again, why not take a short vacation from it? Just think: you could go anywhere in the world!

11
Potpourri

Sometimes I feel lonely in my habit. My husband almost never smokes weed because, as an avid runner, he's averse to sullying his lungs. Very few of my friends still toke up, although many once did. Smoking weed often feels retrograde, slightly seedy. Here I am, alone in my study, rolling up another joint, glad nobody can see.

Then I go online and take comfort in the cannabis community.

🌿

Marijuana is the most popularly used illegal drug worldwide.
— *The Lancet*

Marijuana is beneficial to many patients.
— *Jocelyn Elders, former USA Surgeon General*

Cannabis is remarkably safe. Despite its use by millions of people over thousands of years, cannabis has never caused an overdose death.

— Professor Lester Grinspoon,
M.D., Harvard Medical School

The illegality of cannabis is outrageous, an impediment to full utilization of a drug which helps produce serenity and insight, sensitivity and fellowship.   *— Carl Sagan*

I support legislation amending Federal law to eliminate all Federal criminal penalties for the possession of up to one ounce [28g] of marijuana.   *—Jimmy Carter*

I support decriminalization. People are smoking pot anyway and to make them into criminals is wrong. It's when you're in jail you really become a criminal.   *— Paul McCartney*

I think that marijuana should not only be legal, I think it should be a cottage industry. It would be wonderful for the state of Maine. There's some pretty good homegrown dope. I'm sure it would be even better if you could grow it with fertilizers and have greenhouses.   *— Stephen King*

I've been smoking weed for 44 years, five nights a week. I'm the poster boy to prove it doesn't do you much harm.

— Lee Child

Do you know how many movies I wrote when I was high?
— *John Stewart*

I smoke a lot of pot when I write music.   — *Lady Gaga*

It really puzzles me to see marijuana connected with narcotics—it's a thousand times better than whiskey—it's an assistant—a friend.   — *Louis Armstrong*

Look, I have never made a secret of the fact that I have tried marijuana . . . About 50,000 times.   — *Bill Maher*

I smoked a surprising, a really breath-taking, amount of grass almost every night.   — *David Letterman*

I like to have a little pufferooni at the end of the night.
— *Sarah Silverman*

With each sip comes relief. From pressure, pain, stress, discomfort.
— *Whoopi Goldberg, on vaping for glaucoma-related headaches*

I enjoy smoking cannabis and see no harm in it.
— *Jennifer Aniston*

People don't get mean on weed, don't beat up their wives on weed and don't drive crazy on weed. . . The only down side I can think of with weed is the munchies.   — *Susan Sarandon*

Never give up the ganja.   — *Morgan Freeman*

We are going to do a screening of *The Interview* in Colorado
where I get baked with everyone first, and we can smoke weed
in the theater.   — *Seth Rogan*

Pot is not a drug. It's a leaf.   — Arnold Schwarzenegger

I smoked pot in college and in the Army.   — *Al Gore*

You bet I did and I enjoyed it.   — *Michael Bloomberg*

When I was a kid I inhaled frequently. That was the point.
                                            — *Barack Obama*

    Some other once or present pot enthusiasts are: Maya
Angelou, George Clooney, Stephen Colbert, Miley Cyrus,
Lena Dunham, Art Garfunkel, Hugh Hefner, Caroline
Kennedy, John Kerry, John Lennon, Madonna, Steve Martin,
Brad Pitt, George Soros, Oliver Stone, Andrew Sullivan, Ted
Turner, David Foster Wallace and Snoop Dogg, who says he lit
up in a White House bathroom.
    Queen Victoria, of all people, was probably a user. Her
personal physician of 37 years, Sir John Russell Reynolds,
wrote a paper in *The Lancet* extolling the effects of cannabis.

He used it to treat menstrual cramps, migraine, neuralgia, epileptic convulsions and insomnia. Surely he would not deny his royal patient the benefits of what he called "one of the most valuable medicines we possess."

Many nineteenth-century literary figures also waxed rhapsodic about cannabis, although not for its medicinal effects.

It is quite exquisite; three puffs of smoke and then peace and love.
— *Oscar Wilde*

I felt suddenly that a cloud I was looking at floated in an immense space, and for an instant my being rushed out, as it seemed, into that space with ecstasy.   — *W.B. Yeats*

Your senses become extraordinarily keen and acute . . . In sounds there is color; in colors there is a music.   — *Baudelaire*

When I read these lyrical descriptions of grass (or its derivative, hashish), I take heart. I am, after all, a tiny part of a grand tradition: a great chain of writers who like to get high. But I am also envious. I wish I had what those guys were smoking!

12
Coming Out to Your Doctor

You've seen the question many times. It's on the questionnaire the receptionist asks you to complete every time you see a new doctor. Perhaps you pause for a few seconds, but then you probably answer "No."

The question is some variant of: Have you ever used illegal drugs?

And although you smoke weed, perhaps on a regular basis, and whether or not it is legal in your state, you probably answer "No" because . . . well, it's just easier that way.

You don't want to prejudice a new doctor against you. And what if your behavior becomes part of your medical record? What if your employer or insurance company finds out?

With all the havoc it might conceivably cause, is it really worth coming out to your physician?

I believe the answer is Yes. Of course, it depends upon your boldness and your risk tolerance, but I think you should let your doctor know if you use marijuana routinely.

The insurance companies don't care about your cannabis use: they review charts just to locate financial irregularities. Your employer does not have access to your medical record. And if you're still concerned about information leaking, you don't have to check "Yes" to the infamous question; you can leave the answer blank or even check "No." You will never be charged with perjury!

But when the physician takes a history, you can still be honest with him or her. Let's say you are asked about what medications you take or could take for a medical condition. That would be an appropriate time to discuss your cannabis consumption.

If you like, before discussing marijuana, you might ask your doctor if what you say next could be off the record—not entered into your chart. He or she is likely to turn away from the screen, look you in the eye—and finally pay you some attention!

There are three main reasons to come out to your doctor:

1. Give Your Doctor a Complete Picture of Your Health
Your physician wants to know about anything that might impact your health one way or another. A good medical history includes questions about your exercise habits, vitamin use, diet, and sleep. Regular cannabis use might also be relevant. Your endocannabinoid receptors are getting the very molecules they were designed to receive!

Your physician is likely to read more health studies than you do, and he or she may know the latest cannabis recommendations, or cautions, for a person with your medical profile.

Let's say a patient of seventy is noticing some memory lapses and is worried about dementia. If she confides that she has a history of marijuana use, the physician can assure her that some age-related memory loss is normal and that cannabis is probably not the culprit. The doctor might even allay the patient's fears by citing recent research at the Salk Institute suggesting that THC could actually reduce plaque formation in the brain.

Or suppose a patient of forty is trying to lose weight. A physician might question the patient's habit of toking up every day after work, as cannabis is known to increase the appetite. (That's why it's given to cancer patients undergoing chemotherapy.) Sometimes one needs to hear the obvious from an authority figure.

Cannabis is remarkably free from side-effects, and there have been few reports of cannabis/pharmaceutical drug interactions, so the doctor doesn't need to know about your marijuana use before prescribing you medications. Rather, he or she might prescribe a less powerful dose of, say, a painkiller, because the cannabinol in your system is already providing you with some pain relief from your rheumatoid arthritis.

2. Benefit from Your Doctor's Expertise

You are the authority on what feels right for your body and your mind, but your physician is the expert on health and disease and on the conditions that may ail you. It's good to at least consider what the doctor has to say. You may think you're controlling your glaucoma by smoking weed (which does reduce intra-ocular pressure), but your ophthalmologist may recommend that you supplement your regimen with certain eye-drops. Instead of needing to take them twice a day like most people, because you smoke weed, you may be advised to take them only once a day.

A doctor may be able to warn you that consuming cannabis may interfere somewhat adversely with some common pain medications, such as aspirin, acetaminophen and Darvon. In each case, cannabis, unsurprisingly, increases transient side effects such as dizziness, drowsiness, and confusion, especially among the elderly. Grandma, you've just had your aspirin! Go easy on that vaporizer!

3. Create Teachable Moments

Perhaps you're a high school teacher or a state employee. In certain parts of the U.S., you can't be open about cannabis without jeopardizing your career. You can't participate in the #ComingOutGreen movement for fear of losing your job. But you can be an advocate for legalization on the micro level, one to one, with the people in your life, including your health care providers.

Earlier here I assumed that you have a knowledgeable, cannabis-friendly physician. But perhaps he or she is the opposite: a doctor who doesn't know about (or dismisses) the many medical uses of cannabis, or a doctor who regards pot-smokers as a bunch of stoners. This doctor might still be an excellent physician, so do not storm out in a huff! For a puff!

Rather, this is the ideal time to share the success you've had, say, in using cannabis as an anti-depressant: you can explain that it helps you get more sleep and feel more hopeful. Tell your gynecologist if you've been using pot for menstrual cramps since you were seventeen. If you use weed to avoid migraines, educate your doctor! If your physician gets many such reports, one day he or she might suggest to a patient, "You could try smoking a little marijuana when you get that aura announcing a migraine. Some people say it makes the migraine go away."

Even if smoking weed has no direct impact on your physical health, it's good to let your doctors know that people of a certain caliber (such as readers of this book) are marijuana users. We are not stoners living in our parents' attics and garages. Cannabis is routinely and responsibly used by millions of successful, productive individuals, women and men, young and old.

Before marijuana becomes legal everywhere, both as a medical miracle and a harmless euphoriant, millions of educational encounters need to occur.

Many can take place on the examination table.

13
The Wedding Weed

When my son Simon is the first of the three to get married, I know I want a lot of good weed for the wedding, to be held in California. Since the advent of full body scanners, I'm no longer flying with pot on my person, so I ask Andy, my oldest son, to get some for me. He has a medical marijuana license and can buy the best. As it turns out, he doesn't go down to the dispensary; he gets some from a friend, and it's potent and pungent—ludicrously aromatic. You don't need to smoke it to smell it. Even in its double baggie, it quickly perfumes any room. The red cloth sack which jauntily encloses the baggies becomes a diffuser. Put it in a drawer and the skunky aroma goes into the wood.

The day before the wedding, I smoke a joint with one of Simon's best friends from high school. Smoke provides a shortcut to ease and freedom and nostalgia. I smoke with my nephew. I smoke with my sister. Over the course of several days, people know who to see if they want to get high. They can probably smell it wafting from my handbag.

It's great weed, of course, and I'm high and happy for days. I still have three ultra-fragrant joints left when it's time to go home, and I don't want to leave them behind. I finally put the joints into a three-inch plastic box that holds the balls of wax I put into my ears before swimming. Then I enclose the little box in my bathing cap, wrapping the silicone cap around the box several times. After that, I put the cap in its clear polyethylene storage bag and zip it closed. I put this airtight little packet into a running shoe. Then I put the shoe deep into a metal suitcase. I sniff at the opening. I don't smell a thing. I am safe and the trip goes smoothly.

All this anxiety over three joints! Oh, but it's the wedding weed, and perhaps I will freeze it and we can take it out and smoke it, with ceremony, on their first anniversary.

This doesn't happen. I smoke it all up in the next several days, before my next visit to Ephraim.

14
Saint Bev

The week before Mark and I leave for France, where Mark is running in the Paris Marathon, my mother has an accident and urgently needs someone to care for her. I think about canceling the trip—but then I call a nurse who lives near her in Sag Harbor, who recommends her friend Beverly. Bev, about ten years my junior, has been assisting my mother ever since, although now only part-time.

Saint Bev is how I think of her, because of her easy disposition and intuitive knowledge of what my mom needs. Bev knows that a bedridden patient (as my mom was after her accident) needs a large table by the bed for pills, books, iPad, phone, water, bell, telephone, etc. She knows that my mom loves to cook, so Bev has become a *sous-chef,* dicing onions and parsley, squeezing lemons, peeling garlic and cutting vegetables for later use. Bev has a comfortable SUV and drives my mother to doctors' appointments. Bev is at home on the computer and helps my mother plan trips. Bev sometimes picks up odd useful things for my mother at tag sales and refuses to be reimbursed. Bev helps my mother with her feet, inserting the corn protectors in between the toes and trimming the nails. And she's a good conversationalist, too. Bev visits my mom four days a week, four hours a day, and it's my fervent hope that when my mother needs more help, Bev will be able to provide it.

When my mom turns 90, we have a big party. It's a beautiful celebration on the back lawn leading to the beach, with a classical trio playing Mozart and servers coming around with hot hors d'oeuvres (my favorite food group). After cocktails, the guests gather under a tent for a meal. Then we come inside and tell little stories about my mother, featuring her charm, her intelligence and her genius at making friends. After most people have left, Mark, my sons and some others gather on the hillock overlooking the bay for a sort of after-party. I pull out a joint.

Bev, sitting nearby, produces a vaporizer.

I stare at her in the dark. *Saint Bev is a doper? With professional equipment?*

First I am shocked. Then I am surprised at my reaction. I, of all people, should be tolerant of fellow smokers. But not on the job, part of me insists, not if the job is helping my mother! I answer myself: Bev probably doesn't get high before work. And even if she does, habitual smokers can come down on a dime when they have to—say, for an emergency. I see how I've been brainwashed to automatically think of getting stoned on the job as a bad thing, even though personal experience has shown it can be useful. When I sold advertising space, sometimes on

Friday afternoons I would brainstorm stoned at work.

Bev takes out a lighter from her pocket and gives me a smile. We have a new commonality. But after that night, I no longer think of her as Saint Bev.

15
Coming Out to Your Kids

As a parent, you may have been dreading the question even more than "Is Santa Claus really real?" When your little one asks, "Did you and daddy (or mommy) smoke pot?" what exactly do you say?

It's even worse when your young son or daughter inquires, in a voice of disdain, eyes blinking (oh, yuck), "Do you, like, ever use weed?" Present tense. Here and now. Truth and consequence.

What do you do? Tell it like it is? Lie? Prevaricate?

Where Do You Live?

A lot depends on where you live. If you reside in a state where recreational marijuana is legal, it's much easier to be honest about weed with everybody in your life, children included. Many pot-smoking parents have never hidden their grinders or their bongs, any more than drinking families hide their whiskey or their ice buckets.

People in some states are lucky enough to live the dream

and can be totally open about pot, as if using marijuana were a perfectly safe, natural and unremarkable way to unwind (shh: it is).

What Is Your Job?

Even where legal, however, if you're known as a pothead it might hurt your career or reputation. You don't want little Cristabel lisping to your boss, "Mommy smokes a joint every night before dinner." If you're in the arts or in tech, smoking weed probably won't hurt you professionally, but if you're in education, medicine or law, it probably will. The vast majority of Americans cannot be completely candid about cannabis because of legal, professional, and social consequences, and this affects what they tell their children. These parents must fashion an individualized, age-appropriate response to the question, "Do you smoke pot?"

Little Children

When the children are little, say, under six, it's probably best to avoid the subject by basically hiding your consumption (and accoutrements) from them.

If they don't see it or smell it, your children may not ask you about it for a while. If they catch you in the act, you might choose to evade the issue, "Oh, this? It's an herbal cigarette I sometimes smoke when I get headaches/backaches/stomachaches."

Nothing is more boring to children than adult health issues, and they will likely drift away.

You aren't exactly lying, and, importantly, you aren't asking your child to hide what you do. Asking a little girl or boy to keep a secret is like asking a dog not to chew a bone.

Grade School and DARE

Some grade schools still use DARE, which stands Drug Abuse Resistance Education, a program launched in 1983 by the Los Angeles Police and the Unified School District to teach children about the dangers of drug use. Officers visit classrooms teaching students to resist peer pressure and avoid drug experimentation. That is: "Just say no."

At the height of its popularity, DARE was found in 75% of American school districts and was funded by the US government. In some cases, children are encouraged to talk about their family's drug involvement. DARE has been largely discredited as preventing drug use; indeed, some say it stimulates, rather than discourages, an interest in drugs.

Nonetheless, while its influence has waned, certain districts still participate in the program. If your child is subject to DARE, continued discretion is essential so that Liam doesn't confide to the friendly policeman that daddy sometimes uses weed to get chill. You might consider getting together with other parents to keep DARE out of your school.

Private Morality and the Law

Once children are about eight or nine, they're old enough to learn the difference between private morality and the law. Some laws are bad, and some people resist bad laws. Laws about slavery were resisted by people who sheltered runaway slaves. During World War II, Danes broke the law when they began wearing yellow stars, signaling they were all Jews. Today, environmentalists sometimes gather on private property, or in public places, breaking laws on behalf of their cause.

You might talk about marijuana prohibition, comparing it to alcohol prohibition and noting that both were colossal failures that encouraged criminal activity. You might say that you and millions of people find cannabis helpful in various ways, even though for many years it was officially classified as a Schedule 1 drug, indicating it was harmful, with no medical benefits. Federal prohibition was based on this false premise.

You might tell your kids that for thousands of years cannabis has been used as a medicine and to get people high, without a single overdose. Marijuana is a safe and helpful plant, appropriate for adult consumption, sometimes as an alternative to alcohol or pharmaceutical drugs.

Middle School

As your children get into middle school, you might have teachable moments discussing who benefits when marijuana is illegal and what your state is doing about legalizing cannabis. You might talk to them about marijuana as a social justice issue. Whites and African-Americans use cannabis at comparable rates, but there are 4.5 African-Americans for every white person in New York state prisons for marijuana offenses.

Then there's the fear factor. A few years ago, a teenage boy with marijuana in his pocket fled to the roof of his building with the police in pursuit. He jumped toward the next roof—and fell to his death.

High School

It's unlikely that your children will get to high school before asking you whether you smoke pot, but if that's the case, tell them the truth. High school kids are likely to know friends who use weed, and they themselves may have already tried and enjoyed it. Perhaps they are really asking you about it for a goof! If you can trust your child to be discreet, a policy of honesty is best. Denial will only lead them to distrust you, especially if Jason and Polly have already found your stash, as they probably have.

The Drug Policy Alliance has an excellent online booklet, "Safety First," which offers advice about navigating rocky teenage shoals. You want to offer good advice without being a prude. You want to tell the truth and be a guide, both at the same time. Perhaps you can share a memory of a time you didn't get into a car with an intoxicated driver but called home instead. Reassure Lily once again that you'll always pick her up and drive her home, no matter how late, no questions asked. Safety first!

A Few Caveats

You should tell your child that pot impedes short term memory and learning, so it's stupid to get high before class. You should tell them that the later a person starts using weed or drugs or alcohol, the less chance they will ever be a weed or drug or alcohol abuser. You should tell them that recent studies have shown that the brain continues to develop until a person is about 22. Until then, it's probably best to minimize using psychoactive drugs. This isn't a scare tactic: it's just common sense.

A Happy Ending

If you've been honest about cannabis with your kids, they are likely to be honest about it, and other things, with you. After they graduate from college, perhaps you'll be passing them a joint as you watch the sun go down. Perhaps Dawnette will say, "No thanks, Mom. I'm not really into it." Perhaps Jake will take a hit, exhale, and say, "It's so cool to do this with you, Dad."

16
4:20 on 9/11

Most of us know where we were when we learned about the Twin Towers. I had a job with a medical publishing company in a New York suburb, and I arrived at work a little late. I heard the receptionist say into the phone, "The second tower, too?"

The office was in chaos. Although nobody was sure what to do next, I knew that this was not the time to sell ads for The Journal of Hematotherapy. Everyone was on the phone, trying to check up on their families and friends in lower Manhattan. Their efforts were often in vain because the circuits were overloaded: people were desperate to contact their loved ones and make sure they were all right.

"All right" meant "alive."

In the first couple of hours, many were sure that this was the beginning of a general war. Radio announcers told us, erroneously, that there were eight rogue airplanes. Four had already crashed; what would the other four destroy?

My middle son was at Colorado College near the Air Force Academy, and I called him to say that if the war got wider, he should put his gear in his car and camp out in the hills.

Everything had changed forever. The homeland had been assaulted. The World Trade Center was only about thirty miles away from my house. Thousands of innocent citizens—3000? 40,000? no one was sure—had been killed in a coordinated terrorist attack.

Soon, people were leaving the office for home. For some, because of transportation disruptions, the journey would take many hours. I lived a few minutes away, and I offered to put up anyone who needed it, but in times of crisis, you want to be with your family, not your colleagues. So I went home alone to watch TV and wait for my husband, who would be coming home from his job in Connecticut at six.

It was now around four. I didn't know what to do next. I couldn't watch TV another minute. People kept jumping out of high windows, and buildings kept crumbling to the ground, sometimes in slow motion. Again and again, giant clouds of smoke and debris rose over the ruins.

I needed consolation. I needed communion with nature. I needed to surround myself with beauty. It was a superb September afternoon: sunny, crystalline, 70 degrees. I went to the harbor near my house and lowered my kayak into the water. I paddled away from the harbor patrol and lit up a joint.

Until this moment, I have never told anyone about that joint. I leave it that I kayaked in the harbor, grieving for my country. The harbor is under a flight path, and usually I hear the faint rumbling of planes every couple of minutes, but on this day, all planes were grounded, and I paddled under a silent dome. The sky was royal blue, the water was silver, and two white swans glided by my boat. Solace from nature is respectable; consolation from cannabis is not.

But why not? I'm sure more Valium was consumed on 9/11/01 than on 9/10/01, and we are now learning that marijuana can work as an anti-anxiety and anti-depressant medicine that's safer to the body than any pharmaceutical. Then as now, I did not have a prescription for a psychoactive drug, but I did have my then-illegal stash.

Sometimes pot acts as an enhancer, sometimes as a minimizer, making misery and memory less intense, which is why it is useful for those with PTSD. That September Tuesday, smoking pot did not make everything better. Thousands of people were still dead, and no one knew what the next weeks would bring. But cannabis somehow eased my fears about the future and blunted the horror of the day.

Maybe that's why joints are called blunts.

We all have our own ways to stave off despair. "Whatever gets you through the night, it's all right, it's all right." Now, all these years later, I can finally admit to getting high on 9/11.

17
But Is It Healthy?

After leaving my job selling advertising space, I do my best to expand the little editing business I've started on the side. I love working with words and making writing better, and people say I'm good at it, so I hope to earn a living as an editor. Because most business documents are desperately dull, I believe there's a genuine need for my services in the corporate world; so I call my company Executive Editor, thinking this to be a business-friendly name. My website proclaims, "We do the edit, you get the credit!" I begin a minor marketing campaign, but I do not get many clients. Apparently, most executives are perfectly happy with their prose and see no need to outsource their editing. Apparently, they don't find their own writing to be as tedious as I do. Apparently, I've pitched my services to the wrong market.

A scientist-friend of mine works at a major pharmaceutical company, so I ask him for the name of the communications director and send her my résumé, which I have tailored just for her. Surely they must have material for me to edit. Since

I have, after all, been working in medical publishing, I could even be seen as credentialed, although my job was selling advertising pages in peer-reviewed journals. I am vague about my job on that résumé.

Months go by, and my editing business remains slow. I get the odd novel manuscript to critique or résumé to improve, but I'm scarcely working. Then I hear from Jeanine, the communications director at the drug company. She'd like me to write a short white paper (not edit one!) about biologic drugs. She tells me which researchers at her company to contact by phone and which points I should cover. (This she calls a "backgrounder," a term that makes me smile.) The deadline is weeks away and the compensation is good, so I say yes.

I did not expect to be writing a paper on biologic drugs! I don't even know what they are. I haven't taken biology since high school. Yet my initial ignorance proves no barrier to writing the piece. I begin doing research online. Sometimes a word I don't know is defined by other words I don't know, and I must learn what those new ones mean as well. When I interview the researchers, I say that my piece has to be clear to non-scientists (which is true), so could they please explain things at a very basic level? I write it all up. Before I submit the piece, I vet it with my scientist-friend. He corrects a couple of things, and, quaking, I send it to Jeanine.

Over the next few years, I write some forty pieces for her company.

To preserve memory and foster neuronal connections, older people are often advised to learn a foreign language. I consider life science my foreign language, a way to keep my brain supple. Of course I like the money, but when Jeanine proposes a piece, the real reason I always say yes is to keep my mind alive. Although it's gotten easier, writing these articles remains a challenge, one I perpetually relish.

I am always straight when I interview the scientists, but I usually get stoned to get the piece started and, once again, for the final review.

What is all this pot-smoking doing to my health? I'd like to think it was actually enhancing it, but . . . "What does science tell us?" As if on an assignment from Jeanine, I start looking into the current thinking about marijuana and health.

Reader, be warned! The following is hardly a thorough and impartial review of the field. This is just my quirky summation, no doubt informed by confirmation bias: I desperately want to think weed isn't harmful, because if it is, then I am damaged goods.

However, the overwhelming evidence suggests that marijuana is one of the most harmless drugs ever used. Not one person has died from smoking pot in all recorded history, although eating it has caused two recent ODs. For people who smoke, most of its effects are pleasant and transient.

Nonetheless, even I must conclude that not each of its effects is benign.

The greatest danger faced by pot smokers, especially those over 60, seems to be an increased risk of heart attack, especially for those with incipient heart problems. Toking up can increase heart rate by 40 beats a minute and can cause blood pressure fluctuations, which can temporarily raise the odds of a heart attack.

When I read this, I grow very concerned—until I read on and learn that both exercise and sex are associated with similar short-term heart attack risks. That puts smoking weed into perspective. Sex, sport and smoke are part of living well for me, and I want to keep enjoying them for as long as I can. I'll take the risk with all three.

Another danger, especially for young people, is that marijuana might trigger a psychotic episode or even bring on schizophrenia. Brain scans reveal that after taking THC, the active ingredient in pot, volunteers show reduced activity in the brain area that keeps inappropriate thoughts and behavior in check. (At this point, I regard it as a pleasure to be unbalanced by inappropriate thoughts!) The theory goes: if a person is already fragile, smoking very potent pot might bring on or exacerbate mental illness.

One universally acknowledged problem with pot is its effects on working memory. It's hard to remember things or learn anything new when you're high. On every test of memory, being stoned means you do worse. You should not expect to master Final Cut Pro—or even iMovie!—after getting high.

But unlike drinkers, experienced pot-smokers don't say or do crazy things while high, things they will later forget and regret. Potheads do not black out the way alcoholics sometimes do. They do not wake up in a strange city, beside a beautiful stranger, wondering how they got there. (Actually, that sounds like fun, at least once, but perhaps it happens less often in life than novels and movies would have us believe.)

Another health danger that comes with heavy smoking is

that cannabis lowers sperm count and affects sperm motility. Oddly enough, marijuana doesn't make the little guys slow and lazy: it makes them swim so fast that many burn out before getting close to their goal. Women smokers should know that the THC in their secretions might affect the swimming sperm. So if you're a couple making a baby, it seems wise for both of you to lay off the ganja for a while. (I must confess that Stan and I, in our rank ignorance, did not cut back on weed before conceiving our three sons.)

The most worrisome aspect of marijuana consumption may be its possible lasting effects upon the brain, especially if used before age 25. It has recently been established that the brain goes on maturing until about that time, and, according to the *Journal of Addictions Medicine,* smoking pot may cause impairments "that do not remit with abstinence, particularly if heavy use was initiated in adolescence such that maturation of executive functions was not achieved.. . . These deficits are most evident in tasks that require concept formation, planning and sequencing abilities."

This is a sobering warning, but what if "maturation of executive functions" is achieved early, say at 16? Would smoking at 17 then make a person dopier? My tiny sample suggests not. All three of my sons are remarkably focused, motivated and skilled at long-term planning; each started smoking before he was 20. Still, until the subject is studied more carefully, it seems wise not to smoke much while the brain is still forming.

Of course, it's common knowledge that people in their late teens and early twenties are drawn to risky behavior. Of all possible risks (say, motorcycle racing, sleeping around and going to war), smoking pot is pretty low on the scale.

And what about lung cancer? Marijuana smoke is comprised of some 400 compounds, and users draw it into their lungs and tend to hold it there, even though this doesn't get them any higher than breathing it out like a puff of tobacco. Surely, inhaling and retaining marijuana in their lungs is bad for them, right?

Yet in 2006, the *Washington Post* reported, "The largest study of its kind has unexpectedly concluded that smoking marijuana, even regularly and heavily, does not lead to lung cancer. The new findings 'were against our expectations,' said Donald Tashkin of the University of California at Los Angeles, a pulmonologist who has studied marijuana for 30 years. 'We hypothesized that there would be a positive association between marijuana use and lung cancer, and that the association would be more positive with heavier use,' he said. 'What we found instead was no association at all, and even a suggestion of some protective effect.'"

A suggestion of some protective effect? My heart sings. Could it be that my habit is actually good for me? Some people think THC might kill aging cells and keep them from becoming cancerous. For years, natural healers have claimed that rubbing THC oil on tumors causes them to shrink. Others think it may have an immunoprotective effect. Cannabis may function as an antibacterial; perhaps it also works as an anti-allergen (although not for me). Some studies indicate that it calms Alzheimer's patients and may even retard the progress of the disease.

On its website, the National Organization for the Reform of Marijuana Laws (NORML) states: "Modern research suggests that cannabis is a valuable aid in the treatment of a wide range of clinical applications. These include pain relief, nausea, spasticity, glaucoma, and movement disorders. Marijuana is also a powerful appetite stimulant, and emerging research suggests that marijuana's medicinal properties may protect the body against some types of malignant tumors, and are neuroprotective."

Lest you scoff because NORML is a pot advocacy group, consider what Lester Grinspoon of Harvard Medical School has to say: "Just as penicillin, after its discovery as an antibiotic in 1941, was soon hailed as a wonder drug because of its limited toxicity, its versatility in treating a number of different kinds of symptoms and syndromes, and its limited cost, we believe that marijuana, for the same three reasons, will eventually be hailed as a wonder medicine."

Cannabis as medicine was much acclaimed in the past. In ancient India, it was used to treat insomnia, headaches, stomachaches and pain, and its psychoactive properties were well known. In ancient Greece, it was used to dress wounds and treat nosebleeds. In the Islamic world, it was used for a thousand years as an antiemetic, an antiepileptic, an anti-inflammatory and an analgesic.

Today, medical marijuana is legal to some degree or other in dozens of states, and, anecdotally, cannabis has proved useful for many conditions. Because it's difficult to get funding to do research on a Schedule 1 Controlled Substance such as marijuana, there have been few rigorous studies done on cannabis efficacy, but evidence is emerging that it can help people with a variety of diseases.

Glaucoma is among the most common conditions treated with medicinal marijuana because pot lowers intraocular pressure. Traditional glaucoma drugs do so as well, but pot may have gentler side effects. Glaucoma patients could try augmenting their traditional eye drop regimen with a little pot at night. This will also help them get to sleep.

Insomnia is another condition that has been successfully treated with medical marijuana. While pot's tendency to produce fatigue is usually regarded as an unfortunate side effect, at night this effect may be beneficial. People who use pot to help them sleep usually smoke an hour or two before bedtime, because initially the lively marijuana mind, obsessive yet distractible, may not make them drowsy. After a while, however, the call to sleep becomes inexorable. While you can OD on sleeping pills, you can never OD on a joint.

An important new use for marijuana is in the treatment of movement disorders. A number of families with epileptic children have moved to Colorado, where their children can get a strain of marijuana, Charlotte's Web, which is high in cannabinol and low in THC. In a small study (19 families), 80 percent said their children's seizures were significantly reduced, and some children stopped seizing completely. CURE, a premier epilepsy research organization, is keeping a keen eye on new research into the use of medical marijuana.

Similarly, the National Multiple Sclerosis Society is investigating how an oral cannabis extract can help patients with MS. In one study, muscle stiffness improved almost twice as much in the group taking the Sativex, an oral spray containing THC, as in the group taking the placebo, and "improvements were also noted in body pain, spasms, and sleep quality." For many patients, Sativex "significantly improved spasticity." The catch? Cannabis tended to worsen cognitive problems in the people with MS.

The Parkinson's Foundation is guarded about whether or not cannabis can help alleviate the symptoms of Parkinson's disease, but they note that there are cannabinoid receptors all over the brain, "and these receptors seem to be concentrated in a region important to Parkinson's disease, commonly referred to as the basal ganglia." Structures within the basal ganglia "are some of the most densely packed cannabinoid receptor areas in the human body. . . A drug directed at these receptors might positively influence the symptoms of Parkinson's disease. Indeed many drug companies remain interested in compounds influencing these receptors."

But why look for a new compound? Since these are cannabinoid receptors, no drug will fit into them as perfectly as a cannabinoid. It's the right key for the lock.

A primary use of medical marijuana is as an anti-nausea agent. It's very useful for chemotherapy patients, helping them retain interest in their food—and helping them retain the food as well. As I'm preparing the first edition of this book for galleys, the *New York Times* runs an article in which friends and colleagues recall the life of Bess Myerson. Maureen Connelly, Press Secretary to Mayor Koch, writes: "After declaring her candidacy for Senate in 1980, Bess's doctors found more cancer cells and put her back on chemo. The way I found this out was that I came into the office on a Sunday morning to prepare her for an appearance on a TV program and she was smoking a joint. I said, 'Bess, this is not the best way to prepare. You won't be crisp.' She said, 'Better to be foggy than throwing up on camera.'"

Smoking pot is also helpful for combating nausea and wasting in people with AIDS. In addition, AIDS and HIV patients often use marijuana to alleviate foot pain. Many people with many diseases feel that smoking cannabis is a safer way to reduce pain than any over-the-counter or prescription pill in their medicine cabinet.

A frequent theme among researchers who've determined that cannabis is helpful for one illness or another is their interest in eliminating its "euphoriant effects." As various strains of weed become better studied, it may become possible to remove psychoactive effects of medical marijuana. Strains with a large concentration of cannabinol and little THC might help a person feel better without feeling high.

Frankly, I feel mixed about the idea of stripping out marijuana's pleasure-giving effects. I realize there are populations for whom that will be useful, but as for me, if the medicine comes with a buzz, bring it on!

18
Hot Tub

It must be a measure of my addiction that although pot has repeatedly put me in danger, I still keep on using. Smoking pot has added adventure and terror to an otherwise law-abiding life. I pay my taxes in full and get my car inspected on time. I've paid off my mortgage and I volunteer for the Committee for the Environment. I'm a conservative tennis player and a cautious skier. I'm not self-destructive and I'm not a gambler, but it turns out I will risk a lot for my habit.

Certain things don't go well together for me: alcohol, pot, sugar, the hot tub. Any three of these can make me weak or make me faint, something I often forget. One December evening, I have a glass of wine at dinner. A couple of hours later, I get into the hot tub with a joint and a glass of honeyed mint tea. The water bubbles and froths around me, and after a few minutes savoring my tea, my herb and my hot tub, I find myself blacking out. I haul myself out of the water and flop into a wrought iron chair nearby. The air is cold, and I crave it. Steam wisps off my body and into the night. I spend ten minutes with my head between my knees, trying to get blood to my head. I put on my terry cloth robe. I do not feel better. I try to stand up, sink down on the chair and remain for another ten minutes. I attempt to rise again but collapse to lie on the cold ground, thinking that somehow the ground might give me strength to rise, but it is even worse trying to get up after that. I'm getting scared. I don't think Mark will hear me if I call, for the windows are closed and I'm not strong enough to holler. And it is very cold and I'm on the ground and I can't move.

And then, all at once, maybe half an hour after leaving the hot tub...I can. I slowly get up from the ground and stagger across the patio and up the porch steps and across the porch and into the house, where I fall onto the couch and pass out. Forty minutes later, I have the strength to get upstairs and into bed.

This episode scares the hell out of me, but I tell no one and continue to smoke.

19
Business Trip

For 11 years of my life, I work selling advertising space in biomedical publications. The company office is a six-minute drive from my house, and I negotiate a two-hour lunch break so I can write at home in the middle of the day. My first duty, I feel, is to fiction, and the 40 minutes net I spend in my study after lunch every weekday are the most productive minutes of my life. I write at least 250 and often 500 words every writing session: time constraints make me very efficient, and I slip into whatever novel I am working on without effort and without pot. At three, relaxed and refreshed, I return to the office. There, I work an extra hour at the end of the day to offset my long lunch break and to "contact my Midwest clients at the end of the afternoon"—the rationale (rather than the need to write fiction) I present to management to justify my odd schedule. That last hour, after the others have left and the office is quiet and dim, is another productive part of my day.

My job has many perks in addition to my (non) commute. The sales staff never works overtime or at night (except when we're at conventions, which are usually held in luxury hotels in nice cities), so we never take home any work. Biotechnology in the late nineties and early twenty-first century feels like the most exciting field in the world, and I am thrilled to be part of it, even peripherally and commercially. I meet Craig Venter, French Anderson and Ian Wilmut, editors of journals whose pages I sell. I learn a little about genomics, gene therapy and cloning, partly because these are interesting and promising areas, and also because if I know a bit about them, I can speak with greater authority and sell more advertising pages. I know almost no basic biology, but I am learning something about the latest life science technologies, and I feel my brain expanding.

The perks of the job are great. Then, alas, there's the actual job. I am, after all, in sales: getting clients to like me and offering them new things (a cover-wrap! a gatefold!) so they will increase their business with my company. "Look at it this way," says my colleague Mary. "They have a budget. They have to spend money. So why not spend it on our journals? Why shouldn't they work with those nice ad reps who take them out to lunch and give them such a good deal on their ads?"

Still, sometimes selling makes me feel sleazy.

Marijuana makes business trips bearable. All day, I look forward to the evening joint when I'll be able to unwind. It certainly improves the dinner experience, unless I have to be sharp for a client, in which case I smoke later on. But I don't usually go out at night. Females who travel for business are known to cocoon, and I am no exception. At seven or so I usually smoke in my room, and after a while, I drift down to the restaurant for dinner. Then I go back upstairs for a pay-per-view movie, to which I invariably pass out. No matter the time zone, I always sleep deeply and well.

Occasionally, I travel with a colleague. I always like it when I get to travel with Jill, one of the officers at my company. Seeing each other in the office is difficult because of the hierarchy. It's an unspoken rule: assistants don't have lunch with managers, and managers don't have lunch with officers. People choose people at the same or an equivalent level to be their friends. I am a manager (although I manage no one but myself) and Jill is an officer, but she "gets" me, sees my worth, makes me feel special. And I admire her intelligence, expertise and entrepreneurial drive. Occasionally, Jill and I sneak out to have lunch together, meeting at the restaurant rather than leaving the office together. She and I share the bond of not liking my boss, another officer, a loudmouth and a bully. Jill and I are also women who truly love men, so we have a lot to talk about.

But we probably wouldn't have gotten stoned together except out of town on a business trip. It is, in fact, our last business trip together. We are in a hotel in Chicago, when I suggest we get high. "I have some with me," I say. As if I go anywhere without.

"Fabulous," says Jill. "It's been so long."

I need to get high so I can find a creative way to tell her I'm leaving the company, having been recruited by another, which promises more money and regular trips to India and China. (As it turns out, that company will close its US operations ten weeks after I start working for them, so I end up getting unemployment insurance checks rather than visits to Asia.)

As it happens, getting high does not show me the right way to tell Jill about my promising new job, and I end up simply blurting out the news.

"You're doing so well with us," she says. "Why are you leaving?"

I say, "You may not know it, but I'm turning sixty." She looks shocked; she herself is forty-five and may have assumed we were contemporaries. I continue, "So I'll probably never get another offer like this. I just have to take it."

She nods. "Well, I'm going to miss you."

I miss her, too.

I also miss a client I'll call Nick. I meet him early on in my selling career, at a conference in Phoenix. His company makes software our readers can use, so our journal is a good match for him. Nick is as unlikely a company marketer as I am a salesperson, so we hit it off at once. He is a gay Native American, fluent in Japanese, totally bald; I am a writer with no sales training, out of my depth scientifically—and even ethically. Should I disclose the real circulation of a journal or should I exaggerate, as is the custom? I use the word "readership" a lot because of its vagueness.

Nick and I eat sushi, exchanging tales of our decadent youth and feeling pleasantly subversive. To cement our new bond, we go back to his hotel room and smoke one of my joints. (This item does not appear on my expense report.) It's the end of a long travel day for each of us; after half an hour we are nodding out. I stand up on tired legs and go back to my hotel room.

In the years ahead, Nick takes the back cover of every issue of the journal, and we continue to kid around on the phone. Has smoking dope together really sealed the deal? Somehow, I feel it has. After that joint, we are simply more frank with each other, and once I even tell him how to find the real circulation of any journal that doesn't have the industry-standard "BPA Audit." To satisfy a postal requirement, once a year, certain kinds of journals have to publish the actual number of copies printed. This is usually done in the tiniest print possible, on the most obscure page. I tell Nick that before advertising in any journal (such as journals competing with ours), he should ask to see a copy of that page.

I am surprised no one has ever asked it of me. Surely someone has gone from selling to buying advertising space in scientific journals. (There's an interesting dynamic between sellers and buyers: the latter, of course, hold the power, but the former make much more money because it's harder to sell than to buy.)

The night before a business trip always has me rolling a few joints to slip into a baggie in my bra. I've decided that while there is a remote chance my handbag or rollaway suitcase will get inspected at the airport, there is no chance I'll be strip-searched. I figure this is 100 percent safe. And, indeed, I've flown like this for years. Rolling joints beforehand and allowing myself one per day means I don't have to take along incriminating cigarette papers or a pipe.

So the night before a telemedicine conference, I go to my stash to start rolling. I pull out a cigarette paper—and see, to my shock, that it's the last one in the pack. It's after midnight, too late to buy any more, and I'll be gone for three days. Should I bring some grass in a small plastic film can and try to get papers in a strange city? This seems risky (the key risk being not finding a place to buy cigarette papers), so I decide to roll one very fat joint to last the whole time. I roll it as big as I can, worrying about the strain on the paper. I put the baggie around it. The next morning in the taxi, I tuck the baggie inside my bra. Aloft, I discreetly take it out and put it in my handbag, because body heat makes grass aromatic. I put it back inside my bra as we approach Vancouver.

Vancouver? Yes, I am compounding my flying risk by carrying pot to another country: crossing international borders with a controlled substance. I just can't imagine getting caught, or, if caught, there being major consequences. Getting held up might be a little embarrassing, and I might be late for the conference, but surely the sane Canadians would decline to prosecute a middle-aged American citizen for one single (very necessary) joint. Still, I am uneasy at Canadian customs. Then I see the dog.

A dog! The one thing I haven't thought of. A Canadian customs official is leading a black and brown German shepherd. Rather, it is leading her—in my direction. As it approaches, sniffing the ground, I frantically grope within my handbag for the tiny flagon of perfume I carry with me. I find it and give my neck a spritz. Now the dog is straining at the leash, moving toward me. He slows in front of me, sniffing, and I stare nonchalantly into the distance, heart pounding so hard I'm sure the dog can hear it. I wait for him to bark. One beat, two beats, three. The dog moves on.

I let out a long breath, glad for the perfume. But perhaps the dog isn't trained to sniff out marijuana; maybe he's trained for cocaine or explosives. Or maybe the dog's paraded around just for effect, to make people nervous about smuggling. It's worked. My heart is still beating fast.

To allay my anxiety and celebrate my relief, I need to get high. So as soon as I get inside my hotel room, I take out the very large joint (a mini cigar) I have brought to last the duration of the trip. My room is on the top floor of a high-end hotel, and I am pleased to see that the windows actually open.

It's a purple May evening, and the air is warm and gusty. I take out the fat joint and the lighter and lean my upper body out the window. I thumb the steel, I get a flame, I bring the joint toward it—then somehow I fumble. The joint tumbles from my fingers, and I stare after it in shock as, whirling a little, it starts falling ten stories down. At the fourth or fifth floor, it disappears. I grab my room key and run to the elevator. Downstairs, I dash across the lobby and rush outside the hotel.

What do I think—that on this breezy night I'll find it on the pavement or by the plantings? That I'll just look down and there it will be, my endearingly fat joint, ready to soothe me and smooth me and make me feel good? Why not? It could happen. I search the area: once, twice, again. But there's no marijuana miracle; it's gone. There will be no herbal cocktails in Vancouver, and all because of my clumsiness.

I get through the days of selling. I go without weed. I don't have the shakes or delirium tremens. I survive. But as soon as I'm home I light up. Aaahh. After even a little break, the smoke feels even better, going down my throat, warming up my brain.

20
How to Smoke
Almost Anywhere

So how do I do it? How do I smoke almost every day for 50 years (except when I'm pregnant or nursing) without ever getting busted? Sure, it's easy in one's living room or garden, but what about, say, those bed and breakfasts where hand-lettered No Smoking signs decorate three surfaces in the room? There's no smoke more aromatic than pot smoke, so I have to open a window, push up the storm window or screen and stick my whole head outside before lighting up. I always place a rolled towel to cover the crack under the door to the hall in case the outside air brings a little smoke back into the room After I finish smoking, I leave the window open until the room is aired out.

How do I smoke in a modern hotel with windows that don't open? I go to the bathroom, close the door, turn on the ventilation and stand on the toilet to get the joint within inches of the fan. It's not a poetic environment, but it is pretty safe. But what about the ethics of smoking on a nonsmoking floor? I think it's okay because I smoke only in the bathroom, right near the fan. It's not like the smoke will linger in the carpets or draperies. But what if I fall off that toilet and hurt myself? How will I explain it?

How do I smoke on the street? By rolling a joint almost as thick as a cigarette, so visually it passes for one. I either find a secluded doorway or I look for a stretch of sidewalk with no one approaching from either direction. *Hisss*, the lighter flares, *sssuck*, I take the first hit, and then I walk in a purposeful yet nonchalant manner, toking up several more times before pinching out the roach and putting it in my pocket. Perhaps a pedestrian catches a whiff, but I'm striding along, and the smoke could be coming from anyone. As I get older, I get bolder, because people don't look at me as attentively as they once did. And they don't expect a person in late middle age to be flagrantly breaking a law.

Parking lots are good. So are empty park benches and the ends of suburban train station platforms, such as the one near where I live. The joint, as opposed to the pipe, is essential to my public smoking: a little glass pipe is bound to draw more attention than a seeming cigarette, and the pipe requires lighting and relighting, while a well-rolled joint needs only one flame. I like to think that because I smoke out in the open, the distinctive smell of grass will soon dissipate, leaving no evidence of my mildly criminal act, but this is probably a fantasy.

At music festivals, I slip away behind some trees. On the beach, I crouch by the dunes. At convention centers, I make for the stairwells or the open air. I remember smoking on the stairs with Regina at an MLA convention in New York some forty years ago. I remember slipping outside to get high at a Genome Sequencing and Analysis convention party at Hilton Head. Airports are more challenging, but I rise to the challenge because I love flying stoned, especially for lift-off. Most airports are nonsmoking facilities, so parking lots are the best bet here, especially since most are self-service. Once, riskily, I smoke in an airport ladies room, putting out the joint between each inhalation. Since I inhale almost all the smoke, its aroma is at a minimum. So when I leave the stall, who is to say that I was the smoker rather than the woman in the next stall? At least, that's my reasoning.

What about in a car? Actually, I try not to smoke in a car, and certainly not when I'm driving. Pot makes me an anxious driver: everything seems worrying, even alarming. I sometimes lose my sense of orientation, so at a familiar intersection I might not know which way to turn. Pot also makes me a nervous passenger. If one of my sons drives at more than 30 miles an hour on local streets, I'm grabbing the ceiling loop for stability and wondering why he's so reckless. I don't want the smell of pot to linger in the fabric of the car seats, and the risk of arrest is far greater in a car than in most places. You can get stopped for a broken taillight and get arrested for marijuana possession. So I smoke at home or at my destination rather than en route.

Part of being able to smoke almost anywhere is being able to hide my habit. Sometimes even in my own house I don't want to announce to everyone that I'm smoking *once again*, so

I step outside and smoke on the porch. If it's cold, I stay inside and smoke by the fireplace. With the flue open, the smoke goes right up the chimney. If I'm cooking, I just turn on the ventilation fan and keep my hand under the stove hood. (But where does the smoke vent? Am I infusing my block with marijuana fumes, announcing to this neighborhood of young families that an old pothead lives here?)

After I've smoked, if I want to conceal it, I have a six-step routine. I put eye drops into my flaming eyes and take an ibuprofen, which constricts the blood vessels and makes my eye-whites actually white. I wash my hands with soap and spray on perfume. I brush my teeth and swallow something, anything, such as some juice or a cookie. Then people who don't smoke pot would probably be fooled. Of course, those who know me know I'm high because I smell of toothpaste and perfume—at some random time like 4:20 pm.

21
Nicknames

As with sex and sexual organs, marijuana has a host of synonyms, from the medical to the slangy. It is cannabis sativa or just plain cannabis. It is hemp or herb or, most frequently, weed. It used to be grass or pot. Before that, it was reefer or boo or even boom. Or Mary Jane or just plain smoke. Or sometimes dope, which gives it a dangerous caste, as if it were an opiate. It is bhang if you are from the Indian subcontinent and ganja if you are Jamaican, or aspire to be.

The power of naming is nowhere better illustrated than in the history of marijuana prohibition in America. Throughout colonial and early American history, the cannabis plant was legal. Certain strains of hemp were grown industrially for their fiber, seeds and oil. Other strains of cannabis were routinely used as medicine, often in tinctures.

In 1930, Harry J. Anslinger, a law-and-order evangelist and a racist, was appointed as commissioner of the newly-created Federal Bureau of Narcotics, a post he held for 32 years. He made it his mission to make cannabis illegal, so he called it "marijuana," which was a Mexican slang word for weed. In sensational and unsubstantiated stories of marijuana murder and mayhem published in the Hearst papers, Anslinger demonized cannabis before the hemp industry and the medical profession quite realized what was happening. Anslinger portrayed the plant as an immigrant vice, a lower-class habit and a danger to white America. He stated, "Reefer makes darkies think they're as good as white men…Their satanic music, jazz and swing, result from marijuana use. This marijuana causes white women to seek sexual relations with Negroes, entertainers, and any others."

By calling it "marijuana," Anslinger mounted the most consequential verbal stealth attack in history.

Most words for pot are affectionate. One marijuana website, citing such rarities as "mohasky," "rainy day woman," and "yen pop," lists a grand total of 427 words and phrases for weed. This makes the Inuits' famous 53 words for snow look puny; surely weed has inspired more synonyms than any other substance.

And, as with lovers, there are the personal nicknames. When my sister visits from England, we email about the "valise" I will provide. Like any sane person, she is scrupulous about entering the USA clean, so a luggage discussion is part of every trip. Similarly, on my visits to London, I expect the valise to be waiting in the guest room. I have one friend who talks about "flowers" on the phone. "I need more flowers," she says. "I want a bigger bouquet."

With the octogenarians, we talk about "shoes." They call

needing more shoes. About the same size as the last shoes. They were good shoes, but they're almost worn out. Lately they've been dealing directly with a dealer I introduced them to who makes home deliveries.

I hear that these days they're buying the bud equivalent of Manolo Blahniks.

22
Burning Man

For some time, my sons have been talking about the Burning Man festival, which they've been attending for several years. One year, I decide I must go myself. I was at Woodstock: I want to compare and contrast. My husband, Mark, has a band gig over Labor Day weekend, when "the man burns," so I make plans to go with my subversive friend Jane, also a writer, whom I've known since seventh grade. Her then-partner, Kate, has no interest in Burning Man, but Jane is as curious as I am about the "radical self-reliance" and "radical self-expression" Burning Man promises. I also hope to meet a lot of dopers, some my age.

Burning Man is a weeklong art event which annually attracts some 50,000 "Burners," who camp in tents or recreational vehicles in the Nevada desert. Once you've parked and set up camp, no driving is allowed: everyone rides bikes to get around the encampment, Black Rock City, which is several miles across. Seemingly at random, giant sculptures and play-things erupt from the desert floor. Nothing is sold except ice and coffee, so you have to come with enough supplies for the duration. You have to pack clothes and costumes for 40 degrees at night and 110 degrees by day. You have to have goggles and a headscarf at the ready for the swirling dust storms that descend at a moment's notice. You have to hope that your tent won't blow down around you.

Burning Man selects for the hardy and the physically fit, and Jane and I feel we are probably up to it. We gather it's also for hedonists, and we're probably up for that, too. There's apparently a lot of costuming and a little nudity at Burning Man. Women might wear tutus and brassieres; men might wear skirts and Mohawks. I'm not into nudity myself, but I like to be around it. I start assembling a Burning Man wardrobe. It will be fun going with Jane: we'll be two girls together (girls of 60). I reserve a VW camper to be picked up in a San Francisco suburb. Jane is more practical than I am: she'll know how to make the roof pop up and the stove ignite. And she'll help with the six-hour drive to the festival from San Francisco.

Then Kate's mother gets sick. "She's probably dying," says Jane. "I can't leave Kate alone at a time like this."

What about me? I want to say. You're leaving *me* alone.

She continues, "If something happened, Kate wouldn't even be able to call me." At the time, there's no cell reception at Burning Man. Jane says, "You'll find someone else to go with you."

"I won't," I wail. "It's only three weeks away! People have already made their plans. And not everyone is strong enough for Burning Man."

One friend says, "I'm busy, but even if I weren't, I can't think of anything worse than a week in the desert with a bunch of ravers." Another says, "Not at such short notice, but I'm so flattered you asked. I can't wait to tell my daughter!" A third laments, "I'd do it in a heartbeat if it weren't for my asthma."

So it looks like I'll be going to Burning Man alone. My oldest son, Andy, will be arriving early to help his social group, False Profit, set up its theme camp. (Theme camps are large tents or groups of structures which house dozens of people.) I'm sure I'll see Andy from time to time, but I can hardly camp with him and his friends. I'll bring books and my journal and plenty of food and dope. I'll make friends, I tell myself. I'll be fine on my own in a temporary city of 50,000.

I pick up the VW camper, which is more than 20 years old, in Redmond, California. Its interior is as cunning and appealing as I remember from a camping excursion long ago with my first husband, Stan. There's a little sink and stove and fridge and seats and a table and a comfortable bed. I'm glad I opted for comfort—until I'm on the road and comfort doesn't apply. The camper has a sloppy manual transmission, and it sways in the wind. Cautiously, I take it over the Bay Bridge and into San Francisco, where my three sons live.

The next day, I load up the camper with food and an old bicycle of Andy's, and I set off. I go north to Sacramento, east to Reno and north again another two hours through a surreal, alkaline landscape, beige and brown, with no dwellings or trees. In the far distance, a lake of pure turquoise glimmers, disappears, reappears and is gone. There are no plants at all in

the Black Rock Desert; no bugs; no birds; nothing living. You
don't need insect repellent at Burning Man.

At the festival entrance, my ticket is examined and my car
is inspected to make sure I'm not smuggling in another person.
Then I pull up ahead to the greeters, a man and a woman,
beautiful and half-naked, who beckon me to leave the camper.
When I leave the vehicle, they hug me. I try to relax into their
embrace. When they learn I'm a Burning Man virgin, they
spank me on the butt.

I get back into the camper and creep along, looking for a
place to park that is not too far from a row of porta-potties, yet
not too close either. I also want to be fairly near Center Camp,
for the coffee and ice. Finally, I nose the camper into a good
spot. I manage to get the top of the camper up, even without
Jane, but I can't make the refrigerator work. I'll figure it out
tomorrow.

Now to make myself at home. I take out my stash and
sit on the banquette. I roll myself a number. I wonder what
to do now. The Burning Man website and blog are highly
cautionary, even alarming, warning Burners that marijuana is
illegal in Nevada and that undercover cops can be anywhere,
anywhere at all. It would be a great irony to have smoked daily
for decades—only to get busted at Burning Man. What to do?
Should I hike or bike half a mile to the edge of the city and
to the deep desert, where smoking would be safer? After a
day on the road, I don't have the energy. I decide to smoke in
the camper with the windows closed and the smoke venting
upward through the mesh of the pop-up hatch into the desert

skies.

Never in the next five days do I smell any marijuana except mine. As I pass their tents or campers, people call out, "Hey, would you like a margarita?" or "How about a glass of wine?" Never "How about a hit?" or "Want to share a joint?" To my dismay, alcohol seems to be the drug of choice at Burning Man.

Always, there are beautiful, costumed bodies to ogle, and some of the girls go topless. Some of the men go semi-bottomless, revealing their buttocks. There's almost no live music, but the desert floor pulses to a techno beat. And there are giant art installations to behold, and "mutant art cars" made to look like bugs or boats or spaceships, moving slowly down the roads, amid a hundred bicycles. The sheer spectacle of Burning Man is overwhelming: a vast tent city in the desert, yet a mood of instant intimacy prevails. Strangers are smiling into my eyes and I into theirs. I am sharing an orange with a woman at the librarians' tent. I am moving on a wooden dance floor with two dozen partners. I am walking in the noonday sun toward a yoga class, but again and again I am waylaid, distracted, and suddenly there's a dust storm, and I go into the PolyPride tent to escape it. I don't want to be polyamorous with any of the folks I meet there, so after the dust storm I set off again. The man wears a bright red cotton business suit. He sits on a desk chair by the opening to his tent. He asks "How about some lemonade? With vodka or without?"

I never get to yoga.

That night, I have an anxiety dream about Andy: some

very bad thing has happened to him, and it isn't clear whether he's alive or dead. No one will tell me, and I am desperate. I wake up at dawn in dread. I realize it's a little crazy, but I get on my bike and cycle to the False Profit theme camp. I find Andy's small tent within the compound, and I open the flap and peer inside. It's dark in there, and at first I don't even see the shape beneath the bedding. But it's Andy, very still. Is he even breathing? I creep over and give him a nudge. "Andy? Are you okay?"

He moves, thank God, he moves! He raises his head, looks at me in amazement and says, "Mom?"

"I had a dream something happened to you."

He raises himself to a seated position and says, "Something did happen to me," he says. "I almost got killed."

I stare at him.

He says, "A woman fell on me, from a scaffolding four stories high. I hit the ground, crushed by her weight. I was stunned. But actually, I wasn't hurt. And I probably saved her life by cushioning her fall. She was unconscious for a while, and they got the paramedics for her. But I'm fine. My neck hurts a bit, but I'm really okay."

"Thank God! This dream I had was so intense I just had to come see you. What a relief."

"But mom, you don't believe in that stuff. Precognition, ESP, dreams as messages."

"I *don't* believe in them," I agree.

"So?"

"I don't know. I just had to come see."

Over the next few days, I talk to more people than I ever would have done if Jane or Mark had been with me. I go out dancing most nights, riding my bike to where the music is good, flirting, having fun. Once I see a couple on the playa fucking inside a sculpture of a dinosaur skeleton. They greet me merrily. I'm in bed alone by midnight, while the desert pulses around me. I no longer hope to meet dopers here, for it's not a smoking culture. The young people stay up until dawn, fueled by Ecstasy, no doubt. I manage to smoke my dope (I always do), but I have to smile as I realize I'm more anxious lighting up at Burning Man than smoking a joint at the Hilton.

The next year, I get my doper friend Sophia to come to Burning Man with me, Jane having lost interest in the festival (although Kate's mother is alive and well). Sophia is a writer friend with long dark hair, luminous turquoise eyes and an exuberant personality. With Sophia and I both in it, the VW camper is crowded. She has erected a tent nearby, so we don't feel cramped. We have draped the tent with our various scarves so it looks less REI and more *feng shui*. We want to be comfortable and serene in our temporary dwelling.

Along with our individual stashes of pot, Sophia and I have brought some "pharmaceutical-grade Ecstasy" (his words) one of my sons has scored for us. A considerate child, he has also obtained some kind of antidote, white pills that look similar to the Ecstasy, in case we want to come down. This seems unlikely.

Who wouldn't want to try a drug called Ecstasy? Am I not

of the sixties? And isn't it cool that my son got it for us?

We take the drug on our third day at Burning Man. It is not my first time. I took Ecstasy once before with Mark while we were on vacation on Long Island, but then it just made me feel tense. I felt a low humming, as if something ominous was imminent. Over several hours, this feeling grew increasingly unpleasant—before fading away. There were no other effects. Nonetheless, now, a couple of years later, I have great hopes for our "pharmaceutical-grade" product. Perhaps Ecstasy, and not alcohol, is the real Burning Man drug, so taking it is another link to the people gathered here. I may be older and better educated than most, but we're all in this desert, dressed outlandishly, having fun together, taking Ecstasy!

After lunch, Sophia and I each swallow a little white pill.

"Do you feel it? I don't feel anything!" she soon complains.

"It's only been ten minutes. Give it more time."

"Nothing!" she says a few minutes later. "Let's go out."

"Maybe visit Simon?"

"Sure."

This year, my middle son is at Burning Man with the False Profit contingent. So we get ready to go out. You don't just walk out of your tent or camper at Burning Man; you have to prepare. I get busy packing. In my small brown backpack, I put a bottle of water, an orange, a tin of sucking candies, a dust mask, a long cotton headscarf, sunscreen, Vaseline, eye drops, sunglasses, a long-sleeved shirt and, of course, a joint and a lighter, because—who knows?—perhaps a little dope will set off the Ecstasy.

I wear a cap that gathers light by solar panels on its brim. At night, this light provides illumination. Burning Man is environmentally oriented, so my hat is a novelty hit. Sophia and I set off on our bicycles down a road that will take us toward the middle of the circular encampment, a ring called the Esplanade. When we get there, it's crowded with people and art cars, and I feel disoriented, unbalanced. I do not want to ride the bike, so we push them along. "How are you feeling?" I ask.

"I don't feel anything," she insists. "And you?"

"Uneasy. And weak. Not good."

Sophia looks envious that I'm feeling anything at all. I say, "I have to sit down."

We put down our bicycles, and I sit in the shade of the first structure I see. This happens to be opposite a huge geodesic dome in which fierce looking men are swinging from ropes to fight each other. I have collapsed near the worst possible place to do so at Burning Man: the biker theme camp MegaDeath. We are getting hostile looks from men in black leather. Sophia says, "We should go, Cathy." She hoists me up, but I can't manage even guiding my bicycle, so we lock it there and move on. It's just a few hundred yards in the desert sun to the False Profit tent, but it seems like a mile. Finally, we're entering the airy tent, with its curtains of saffron and red. Once within its sanctuary, I sink down again. My legs are rubber and will not support me. Someone goes to see if Simon's at his tent site. Sophia says, "So you're okay now?"

"Yes, if I don't have to move."

"I have to go," she says. "I'm restless. Maybe it's the drug.

See you later."

I watch as she leaves the tent, amazed that she has all this energy while I have none at all. And I'm getting that feeling of ominous immanence again.

Soon, Simon and his then-girlfriend appear. From my huddle on the floor, they seem to loom above me. From this angle, and because she's wearing a loose vest over nothing, I can see that his girlfriend has pierced her both nipples, which makes me feel faint.

"Mom? Are you all right?"

I tell him I can't move because of the Ecstasy. He grins. "Well, I've just taken all these mushrooms." He plops down beside me. His girlfriend fades away. "Why don't we just stay here for a while, and then I'll walk you back to your campsite."

"Do you like Ecstasy?" I ask.

"Once in a while," he says.

"I'm so disappointed! I don't feel ecstatic, only tense. And paralyzed. I simply cannot move my legs."

"That's funny," he says. "Most people like to dance when they're on E. You just have to be contrary." Big grin.

"I guess."

In an hour or so, I manage to get up. Simon gets my bike and pushes it with us to the camper.

The next day I'm not feeling much better. Sophia still feels restless, so we both decide to take the antidote. That afternoon, we'll be reading short stories at Center Camp, and although our audience may be on drugs, we ourselves don't want to be. So we take the little white pills, but they don't seem to be working. In fact, I'm feeling somewhat tense again. And just like that, we convince ourselves that we've taken the wrong pills, more Ecstasy instead of the antidote. We start moaning, "Oh, no!" "How could this happen?" "Please, no!" "Oh, God!" Then I find the clear packets we just opened and study them. Surely they're a different shape than the ones we opened yesterday, aren't they? We're probably fine. And to ensure that we're really fine, we smoke a joint, and that seems to work; we're mellow again, back to normal.

Yes, it's come to that. High is the new normal.

23
Celia

Three years before my first trip to Burning Man, I lose my best friend. I don't lose her to death or disaster or dementia: instead, she tells me our friendship is over. On the phone. After decades, and after no particular incident. Celia has decided that she doesn't want to know me anymore. Almost ten years later, I still feel the pain.

Our friendship goes back to our freshman year at Brooklyn College, when the dean of the Scholars Program fixes us up, as it were. As soon as I am admitted to the Program, after my first semester, the dean says, "You must meet Celia. You two will really get along." So he puts us in the same English tutorial. Once a week in the cafeteria, the two of us get together with our handsome professor, who chain smokes and looks soulful as we discuss the Transcendentalists.

Celia is a tall, striking girl with straight brown hair that falls in a glossy curtain to her waist. She is smart, articulate, vivacious. We both live for books and boys, and soon we are having a glorious friendship, talking, talking, talking. Together we are quite the duo, attracting guys because of my breasts and her elegance—and that amazing hair. It's so long I once see a guy hold the bottom of it, as if it was the fringe on a shawl, and she doesn't even notice.

Celia has a brother named Michael. He plays in a jug band by the wall opposite the library, and I have a crush on him, which I hide from Celia. I know he isn't going to classes because he is always in blue jeans, which are not permitted in the classroom. Celia lives two blocks from campus, so I am often at her house and get to know the family. Mother, father, daughter, son: they never pass each other without exchanging hugs and pats and kisses. I think it's great that she has such a happy family. When Michael comes into the room, I get animated and self-conscious, hoping that he'll notice me, which he finally does. We hide our one date from Celia (his dating her friends has been an issue before), so she never knows how much I grieve when he doesn't call again after what is, to me, a magical evening.

Celia and I spend two years as best friends at Brooklyn College. Then, in 1965, Celia transfers to Berkeley, where she finishes college, and I spend my junior year at the University of Sussex. Celia and I return to New York in our early twenties, and we both get married, at ages 22 and 23, in successive months. After a couple of years, her marriage breaks up and she moves to Greenwich Village. Soon, I move there, too. She is teaching English, working in the public school system like her parents, and I am writing novels and having babies. She has a brief affair with our old English professor. She dates a lot of guys, all of whom play guitar well. I tease: "What do you do? Hold auditions?" In her late thirties, she leaves to get an MA in drama at the University of Michigan. There she meets George. Just in time, she thinks, to finally have a baby. Only it doesn't work out that way; incredibly, after six weeks, they split up. Celia is now at loose ends. Nothing keeps her in Michigan, and she doesn't want to return to New York with its bitter winters, so she goes to Sarasota, where her parents have moved. She starts a program that integrates local theaters with the schools, and I admire her for creating her own job. It doesn't pay much, but she doesn't need much. Somehow, through her parents' generosity and savvy, she has a nice little income. "They give their money, and mine, to this guy," Celia says. "And he always gets a good return."

"Lucky you."

"Perhaps one day it will all disappear, but for now it's terrific."

I visit her several times in Sarasota. It's a cheap winter vacation: she always lives in large, appealing spaces with guest bedrooms. But things are not as easy between us as they once were. Sometimes she's in AA (although I've never seen her drunk), and meetings are the focus of her day. At other times, she drinks some wine at night. This doesn't strike me as alcoholism: after all, I smoke some pot at night—and often in the afternoon as well.

"It's not the same," she insists. "You're not an addict. You don't need it."

"But I do," I say, lighting up. I offer her some, but as usual she shakes her head. She doesn't like the marijuana high.

"You have it easy," she insists. "You like pot and you smoke it. No problem."

"Why is it different with you and your wine?"

"I feel bad about it. I try to stop. And I can't."

"How do you know I don't feel bad about it? How do you know I haven't tried to stop?"

"Have you?"

"Of course."

She looks skeptical. And we're locked into our new dynamic: her insisting upon her unhappiness or craziness while dismissing any of my own. She tells me her seemingly happy family was really dysfunctional, with a domineering father and a pathologically passive mother. She thinks I've always had it easy. "But Stan left me," I protest. "He walked out on me and the kids. That wasn't easy."

"But it was," she says. "You bounced back. You met Mark. You ended up happier."

"That was mere luck. And what about my so-called literary so-called career? Now I don't even have an agent."

"You've had several novels published," she says. "You'll get another agent."

"It's not just the agent. It's about how hard I've struggled and how miserable it is to see other, inferior authors being praised by the critics or having bestsellers. While I remain obscure and ill-paid. I feel too old for that."

"Writers always complain about their careers," she says. "It's an affectation."

"When famous writers complain it's an affectation," I say. "Like when Solzhenitsyn complains he got the Nobel Prize because of the subject of his books and not the style. But I'm not famous, and I have every right to my heartbreak." I say it lightly, but "heartbreak" feels like the right word. I thought that by my fifties I'd be at least a minor novelist, getting asked to contribute to major publications—but that hasn't happened. Since I don't have the glamour of debut, it's getting harder for me just to get published. My batting average with novels is exactly 50 percent; there are five novels in the drawer, by which I mean my hard drive.

Celia doesn't hear me; she's decided my problems don't rate. What happened to our easy understanding, our empathy for each other?

The following summer, we arrange to meet at the Rhythm & Roots folk festival in Rhode Island, where Mark is playing with his band, the Zydeco Hogs. Zydeco dancing is a little like jitterbug or swing, but to a different rhythm. The music, from Lafayette, Louisiana, is lively and infectious, and at a zydeco dance, almost everybody smiles. Celia has taken up zydeco dancing in Florida, and because she doesn't want to be without a partner, she has come to this music festival with Karl from Tampa. On the phone, she tells me that she doesn't much like him, but he's a good dancer. Karl looks like a Hell's Angel, menacing and uncouth, with a scar near his thin, twisted mouth. I'm surprised that she has committed herself to his company for several days, as if she couldn't get a partner on her own. Alcoholic or not, unhappy or not, Celia is very good-looking.

And she's drinking again: she holds two large plastic cups of beer on a tray. Maybe this will help break down her reserve. For she is distant with me, dismissive. She and Karl dance with abandon, but there's something fixed about her grin, and her movements are forced and mechanical. I hope we'll get a chance to talk, but she insists on dancing every number, and when there's a break for dinner, Mark and I lose track of her and Karl. Is she avoiding me? What have I done?

After dinner, I spot her in the crowd and tell her that one of my favorite singer-songwriters, Slaid Cleaves, is about to perform. I'm very excited. "You have to hear him, Celia. He's wonderful."

"No, I'll just stay at the dance tent. I came here to dance."

"Yeah, but . . ." In the face of her indifference to my enthusiasm, my spirit fades. If your friend doesn't care about your likes and dislikes, doesn't want to know what makes you happy, is she really your friend? Mark and I go up the hill to hear Slaid, who gives a terrific performance, as usual.

The next afternoon, Mark's band plays at the dance tent at two. But although she "came to dance," Celia doesn't show up. I see Karl and ask about Celia. "She's not feeling so good," he says with a wink, as if being hung over is somehow endearing. My feelings are hurt, though. You'd think she'd want to hear my husband play. As always, the Hogs put on a fabulous show. You cannot hear their music without tapping your feet or shaking your hips: they are my favorite zydeco dance band. Alas, I can never dance to their music with my favorite partner, who's onstage with his squeezebox. He's festooned with Mardi

Gras beads, and his black shirt shows off his muscled arms. When he's onstage, I sometimes pretend I don't know him, so I can appreciate him objectively. As if . . .

We leave Rhode Island that night without seeing Celia again. I can't understand her bizarre behavior. I wait for her to call and apologize. Weeks pass, then months.

Finally, after almost a year, I call her.

"Oh, Cathy," she says.

There's real regret in her voice, and for a moment I think she's sorry about how she behaved. I am eager to forgive her, because how many old friends do we have?

"I've been thinking," she says. "And I've made a decision. I don't like our friendship. I don't want to be friends with you anymore."

"But what have I done?"

"It's not what you've done," she says, "but who you are."

"Who I am?"

There's silence.

I softly hang up the phone. I can't change who I am. I've been wholly condemned. She never wants to see me, ever again.

The pain lasts and lasts. I can't understand why she's done this. I wake up in the night feeling hollow. Why doesn't she want me in her life? Won't she miss me? Will she talk about me to her shrink—or don't I even rate enough for that?

"She was very cruel," says my mother. "There was no need to treat you like that. But I'm not surprised. I never trusted Celia."

"You're just saying that to make me feel better."

"That's not true. Right from the first, I thought there was something artificial about her. Her smile was too wide. She seemed false."

"But why would she do this to me?"

"Probably envy. She's always wanted children, and you have three. You say she never found work she really likes, while you have your writing and editing."

"Well, mom, it shouldn't be like that. And anyway, there are things about her that I envy." She's multi-orgasmic. She has beautiful hair, skin, and nails. She has financial security.

"Try to get over her," my mother advises.

I can't. Celia's gone from my life, but not from my heart. She doesn't want to be my friend. She doesn't want to see me or hear from me *ever again*. I repeat these words to myself at least once a day, but for years they do not lose their sting. When I think about Celia, shame corkscrews through my chest.

Friendship is central to our lives, but how often do you read about the misery of a broken friendship? I can think of only one book with this theme: Shelby Hearon's *Life Estates*. Mark tries to console me, but he's not as close to any friend as I once was to Celia. Still, he sees how unhappy she's made me. He says, "Whatever her issues, she shouldn't have treated you like that." He feels my sadness almost as keenly as if it were his own.

Years go by. I realize that because she lives a thousand miles away and has a common last name, I'll probably never hear anything about my old best friend again. But I am wrong. One of my neighbors starts dating someone named Jeff. They go up to his parents' summer colony, which is where Celia's parents had a house. When I meet Jeff, I ask if he knows Celia, and it turns out he knows her well. He says, "In fact, I just saw her."

"You just saw Celia!" Everyone else in the room fades away. "She used to be my good friend." I hear the pathos in my voice. "How's she doing?" I can't help adding, "How does she look?"

"She looks fine," he says, "she always does. But she's not doing so well."

"How come?"

"All her money was with Bernie Madoff."

Mark, overjoyed, shouts "Yes!"

"Not only that," says Jeff, "but since she got such a great return for so many years, they're going to 'claw' that money back."

Mark can't help himself: he jumps up and pumps his fist in the air. This is what Celia never had: someone who always has her back. Maybe that's why she can't stand to see me.

"You're such a frat boy!" I tell him.

"As long as I'm *your* frat boy," he replies. "Forget about Celia."

But I can't do that. I still miss her. To this day, I wonder if I could have done anything to preserve our long friendship. I sometimes think if we could have smoked pot together, or if she was the kind of person who liked getting high, then everything might have been different. But maybe that's just a pipe dream.

24
Smoking Kif with
Paul Bowles in Tangier

Perhaps I agree to co-produce the film so I can say, "I smoked kif with Paul Bowles in Tangier"—but it's not so easy to slip this into general conversation. For one thing, few people know what kif is. For another, not many people have heard of Paul Bowles. I joke that the problem with fundraising for a film about him is that half the funders haven't heard of him—and the other half have. Paul Bowles, the American writer and composer, has a somewhat sinister reputation based on the violence in some of his stories, his self-exile to Tangier and the fact that drugs, principally kif, play a significant role in his fiction, a key reason for my interest in the project. Hundreds of novels, both comic and tragic, are soaked in alcohol; I prefer books that are cannabis-infused, for I am comforted to read fiction about lives where weed plays an even larger role than it does in my own.

Then there's the matter of Paul's marriage to Jane Bowles. Each was gay, and they rarely lived together, but they were deeply involved in each other's lives. When Paul stopped composing music for Broadway plays and began writing fiction, Jane may have felt he was invading her turf, for she had just published *Two Serious Ladies*. The international success of Paul's first novel, *The Sheltering Sky*, seems to have drained Jane of further ambition. As we interview various literary scholars, we learn there are "Jane people" and "Paul people."

Funding remains a problem, for in the late eighties, documentaries are shot on film and are very expensive to produce. Film equipment is heavy and difficult to operate, and a skilled crew is costly. So are lab fees. It's not easy to raise $200,000, which our documentary will ultimately cost, for a film about a relatively obscure writer and musician.

Still, Bowles is in many ways an ideal film subject: charismatic, enigmatic, handsome and articulate. He lives in a beautiful city and takes us to the most picturesque spots: to the Roman Road, to the high cliffs, to a tangle of streets in old Tangier, to a lush garden behind an iron gate, whose hinges groan expressively as he pushes it open. Bowles has known some of the most interesting people of the twentieth century and does hilarious imitations of Gertrude Stein, W.H. Auden and Tennessee Williams. He recalls incidents involving Leonard Bernstein, Peggy Guggenheim and William Burroughs.

To tell you the truth, Burroughs gives me the creeps. I can't stand, or understand, his writing; he killed his wife in a game of William Tell; and he looks like he just stepped out of the grave. So when my friend Regina proposes Paul Bowles as a film subject, I say yes—with one condition. "I don't want

William Burroughs in the film." She agrees. Later on, I realize my mistake. Burroughs may be ghoulish, but he's certainly amusing, and including him would have added an entertaining element.

Paul Bowles is about to turn 80, so our pitch to funding organizations goes: "We want to document Paul Bowles, an American original, while he's still alive." We say, "We want to record his life for posterity." Then we start to learn about other Paul Bowles documentaries. This is before the Internet, and there's no central repository of information about films produced or in production, no database to consult. Bowles himself has no telephone. So it's almost by chance that we learn about a twenty-year-old American documentary about him, and a five-year-old Dutch film about him, and an hour-long BBC interview with him. After we shoot him for a week in Tangier, as we are putting our equipment into the van for the last time, a Japanese camera crew starts climbing up the stairs to his apartment.

When we finally finish editing our 57-minute film, I joke that we could hold a Paul Bowles Film Festival, with movies from around the globe. Perhaps every country, no matter how small, has its own Bowles documentary. Bowles maintains that he hates being interviewed, but the documentary evidence is otherwise. In fact, he even plays a role as on-screen narrator in the Bertolucci movie of *The Sheltering Sky*.

Naturally enough, considering my involvement, our film, *Paul Bowles: The Complete Outsider,* is the only Bowles documentary to give cannabis its due. He takes us to the

Café Haffa, on the cliffs overlooking the Mediterranean Sea, where young men pass the hash pipe to each other. We film him talking about how he composed the scene of Port's death in *The Sheltering Sky* after eating *majoun*, a marijuana jam concoction. He talks about preferring pot to alcohol, while smoking a kif cigarette.

When we turn off the camera, Regina, Bowles and I smoke kif together. It's a bright, subtle high, not heavy like the Mexican grass I'm used to. We smile a bit; we don't say much. Later on, we film one of his good-looking Moroccan assistants preparing kif in the living room, rubbing the plant through a fine screen to get a golden pollen-like powder, which has a higher level of THC than ordinary weed.

To distinguish it from the myriad other Paul Bowles documentaries, we start saying ours is the "sex and drugs Paul Bowles film," because we also address his homosexuality, although not with our subject, who is so old-school we dare not broach the issue for fear of inducing an on-screen heart attack.

The film takes years to finish, but ends up doing well, with a New York opening at the Museum of Modern Art, a theatrical run of 20 cities, distribution on the Sundance Channel and wonderful reviews. This has little to do with our stoned brainstorming and a lot to do with Bowles, a legendary writer with an inimitable mystique, and our crew, especially a masterful cinematographer and a brilliant film editor.

Just before we leave Tangier, while I'm still upset about the Japanese crew, I go to a small shop to buy one of those round brass trays that dangle by three chains connected by a ring so you can carry three cups of coffee suspended by your finger. The store doesn't have the tray I want. The shop owner asks if I need any batteries, special Moroccan batteries. I'm puzzled. "Come back here, I'll show you," he says. I'm not aware that batteries vary from country to country. He takes me to the inner room, opens a drawer, and I see a large chunk of hash. "Do you need this?" he asks. "Or a smaller piece?"

Sold in New York, that chunk could pay for ten minutes of film. I shake my head regretfully, sorry I haven't wandered into this shop on the first day of the shoot, and not the last. I would never bring drugs, not even half a joint, back to the USA. Still, I'm pleased that he opened the drawer—flattered in my forties to look like the kind of woman who would buy Moroccan batteries.

25
Stoned Identity

So why am I so pleased when people assume I smoke weed? It's always gratifying to be understood at a glance, but my pleasure goes well beyond that. What is the identity smoking pot confers, or that I think it does? It certainly is prominent in how I define myself: I am mother, writer, wife, American, doper, Jew, dog-owner, kayaker, flirt—perhaps in that order. What pleasure does the doper label bring me? Why do I always hope a new friend smokes pot? What traits does smoking weed suggest—at least to me?

Perhaps throughout our lives we remain attached to the fashions, music, hairstyles and assumptions popular in our youth. When I start getting high at 17, pot-smokers are mainly unconventional, creative people. This is surely not true today, yet the prejudices and assumptions of that earlier time still linger. By the late seventies, high school dropouts and PhD students, bikers and ballerinas, rednecks and bluestockings, soldiers and stockbrokers, gangbangers and trust-fund brats—everybody's getting stoned (although, then, as now, it's mainly young black males who are going to prison for possession). Smoking pot has become an easy and common way to feel good, without the downsides (aggressiveness, hangovers) of drinking alcohol.

By the eighties, cocaine is in fashion, but it holds no interest for me because of the expense and the effects. I don't want to be any more wired than I already am. For me, the first few minutes after snorting cocaine I feel like I'm waking up on a nice day, a *really* nice day. The next hour I'm a nervous wreck, with chattering teeth and a racing heart. I feel both tense and tired.

Although I think of myself as a drug-taker, outside the dental chair there's only one drug I take—and, hey, it's not really a drug, it's an herb!

When I move from Greenwich Village to the suburbs and get a corporate job selling advertising space in medical journals, I become increasingly conventional to the outward eye, and pot becomes increasingly important as a signifier. It means that although I have a business wardrobe and know the jargon of my sector, I'm still challenging boundaries, still open to joy.

To this day, when I learn that someone smokes weed, I like him or her more and imagine us getting high together. I think it's likely we share a "stoned sensibility," which I associate with good humor, easy laughter, sensual intensity and imaginative inquiry—often to the point of absurdity. Stoned conversations are sometimes deeply philosophical and sometimes deeply trivial. They are rarely belligerent or competitive, although they can be fatuous and dull when people can't remember what others have said—or the beginning of the sentence they are now trying to finish.

Getting stoned encourages honesty and humor. It offers a shortcut to intimacy. It feels pleasingly decadent—still, after all these years. I smoke pot, therefore I'm still young, still a rebel. (I know this is ridiculous, but I've vowed to be honest here.) I'm convinced that pot-smokers have a special appreciation for whimsy, wordplay and the works of M.C. Escher. Potheads tend to be gentle, low-key, unstressed. I don't know which comes first: the sensibility or the pot-smoking—or whether one shapes the other. I do know that if a man approached me down a dark street, I'd be frightened if he was holding a bottle and relieved if he was smoking a joint.

26
Smoking with the Kids

I begin this chapter with some hesitation, because I know it will alienate many readers. For surely it's taboo to smoke pot with your kids—yet I've been doing it since they were 18. I do not introduce them to grass, but when I learn that they're routinely smoking pot with their friends, it seems silly to deny ourselves the fun of getting high together just because the neighbors would be shocked. If we'd been a drinking family, surely I'd be serving them cocktails at this age. Instead, I ask if they want to join me on the porch for a smoke (I try to keep the house smoke-free, unless it's very cold outside). They say yes about half the time, which seems about right to me. They like grass quite a lot, but they aren't dependent on it.

There are a few years when I hide my habit from the children as best I can. The D.A.R.E. program, run by local policemen, is propagating antidrug propaganda in the schools, and I don't want Jerome, the youngest, blurting out that his parents smoke pot. What if they ask? He might feel obliged to be honest. He is already highly principled, and in the second grade, much to my surprise and with no input from home, he refuses to participate in Columbus Day celebrations because of his sympathy for Native Americans.

When Jerome is eight, his father leaves me for another woman. I am devastated. Yet three months later, toward the end of our trial separation, I'm not sure I want Stan back. By then I've met Mark. My indecision makes me crazy, my feelings strobing back and forth even as I breathe. Sometimes when I inhale I want Stan back and when I exhale I don't. I go down to the bottom of the garden to smoke and calm down. "I shut the kids out and get high," I tell my sister on the phone. She scolds me. "That's just wrong! You have to be with them." This shames me into smoking less, and Stan and I prepare to live together again.

As we negotiate his return, Stan says that before he comes back I have to agree to some rules. For one thing, he wants me to think before I speak. *Rules?* When he should be down on his knees for letting his affair imperil our family? That does it. I decide I don't want him back yet. I want to get to know Mark better.

Five years later, Mark and I are still together, though not yet married. We take a trip with my three sons to the Grand Canyon. It's our first family vacation with Mark. Throughout the trip, Jerome is temperamental and cranky. At one point, he refuses to get out of bed so we can get an early start from the motel. He puts the pillow on top of his head and lies there like a lump. Andy says to Simon, "Shall we?" and Simon says "Yes!" The next thing I know, Andy has grabbed Jerome's arms, Simon has taken his legs and they are hoisting him to the bathroom. Mark and I stare at each other, wide-eyed. We wouldn't dare do anything like this. They dump him, clothes and all, into the shower stall and turn on the water.

"Hey!" yells Jerome.

"Time to get up," says Andy.

"I hate you!" shrieks Jerome.

Mark and I are doubled over laughing.

We drive several hours before we reach the North Rim. We take our first hike into the canyon. It is spectacular, every bit as magnificent as we had hoped. It is a landscape like no other: from the top, almost as flat as a desert, with the horizon far away and deep fissures going down. Looking down, there are jagged walls of red and beige and purple, layer after layer, receding into the distance From time to time, Mark and I loiter behind the others to take hits off a joint before gawping anew at the views. As I will later learn, my oldest sons, Andy, 24, and Simon, 19, are also finding ways to sneak off together and get high as we hike. So it's only Jerome, 14, taciturn and hostile, who isn't high in the Grand Canyon. Now he's in a bad mood because we insist that he wear his hat to protect his head and neck from the sun.

His bad mood lasts approximately two years, and then one day it vanishes completely. And suddenly Jerome is helping me out in the kitchen and showing me his essays and jokingly trying to sit on my lap after dinner. I feel like I have my son back.

Mark and I have different theories about this sudden change. "He's getting high," I say. "He's getting laid," Mark says.

It turns out we're both right. He has a wonderful girlfriend, and he sometimes smokes pot with his friends. He confesses later that he occasionally takes a little dope from my supply, from whatever hiding place I am currently using. He calls it "the mother lode."

We take a car trip to look at colleges. We have so much to say to each other, we miss an exit. We are having a rollicking time. A few hours later, after touring a campus, we pull into a nearby motel and get stoned.

Now here I must interject a note from 2015. Recent studies indicate that young people's brains continue to mature until their early twenties and that pot may damage executive function development. If this research holds true, of course it was wrong of me to share joints with my kids when they were 18. However, I haven't noticed lack of executive function in any of them, certainly not in Jerome, who is a founding member of a large international organization and works long hours at a complicated job.

Back at the motel during the college tour, we lie on the twin chenille-covered beds, feeling mellow. "Do you see that?" Jerome asks, pointing to a corner of the ceiling. A bit of dust is caught in a cobweb there, moving back and forth as the air from the heater churns sluggishly. For some reason, that trapped particle, fluttering here and there, starts making us laugh, and the breeze from our laughter makes it jiggle more. Soon, we are hysterical, as if this were the funniest thing in the world. We can't take our eyes off it. "Do you realize, mom," he gasps, "we're sitting here watching some dust?"

"No, no," I yell. "Stop. I can't stand it." I have a stomach ache from laughing. I cover my ears with my hands so I won't hear him, and I close my eyes so I won't see that most hilarious of all things, the bit of dust, because truly I am worried that I will somehow burst from laughing. Or maybe only pee.

Jerome recalls this somewhat differently. He remembers the cobweb as being just above a horizontal vent. And when we see it, we start talking about how the cobweb makes invisible air currents visible. We're suddenly obsessed with this idea, he says, "in that stony way people sometimes get" and decide to construct tiny paper sails. We tear up strips of paper, sized and shaped to ideally catch the low breeze of the vent, and tie them with thread. Then we watch, ultra-satisfied, as they merrily flutter in the breeze, making the invisible visible.

I prefer his version, as it shows us to be somewhat philosophical and even scientific.

What a time! Would it have been somehow better if we'd had the laughter without the pot? That seems like the wrong question, for we wouldn't have been drawn to the dust in the web if we hadn't been high in the first place.

27
Urban Farmer

We are driving on a road through the potato fields of Long Island when my friend Anne tells me what she's been doing for the last several years. I'm so surprised I almost drive the car into a ditch.

Meeting at the University of Sussex in 1965—our dorm rooms adjoin—Anne and I quickly become friends. She is a highly intellectual Canadian doing an MA in philosophy. I am a girl from Brooklyn College, spending my junior year abroad. She is tall and beautiful, with straight, strawberry-blond hair and a subscription to the *New Statesman*. I feel she has read every important book in the world, and I am in awe. I'm especially impressed by her boyfriends, who are all very interesting and articulate and homely. That she pays little heed to male beauty is a quality I admire without being able to emulate. One of her boyfriends went to public school with a member of The Who, and when the band comes to play at a university dance, he brings them to tea at Anne's. But her room is too messy, so they all troop into mine. At the time, I think they're silly because of how they sing "My G-g-g-generation," so I'm not impressed.

Anne and I never smoke pot together at Sussex because she doesn't like the effects: grass makes her uneasy. She prefers wine, and these days I always have plenty around when she visits. She probably drinks as much as Celia, but doesn't seem in the least troubled by it, and she would hoot at the notion of going to AA.

Once, when we are in our thirties, I persuade her to try marijuana again, and I bake us some pot cookies. Perhaps I haven't properly mixed the batter, because a couple of hours after ingesting two cookies, Anne cannot move and is miserable. Witnessing her distress, I vow never to eat cannabis again, a promise I have kept. You cannot control your high when you eat pot, and the effects seem to last much longer. As for Anne, the cookies convince her that cannabis is altogether wrong for her constitution.

So we're driving through the potato fields when Anne says, "You know, I've been growing pot in the attic."

"What?" The car veers; I straighten it.

"It's good money," she says.

"But you, of all people, . . . You don't even like getting high."

"That's true," she admits, "but it helps me get to sleep."

"I can't believe this," I say. "How much are you growing?"

"Eight sensi plants with four harvests a year."

"You sound so professional."

"I think of it as just another craft," she says. "I provide an

artisanal product." After MAs from Sussex and Oxford, Anne
has left the academic life and become a craftsperson, initially
specializing in old pottery and presently fashioning exquisite
gilded mirrors and picture frames. I cannot fathom her being
part of the marijuana supply chain.

It all begins with a man called Jay. At the time, Anne
is renting out part of her London house to her friend Liz.
She and Liz, both single, have a crush on this fellow, Jay, a
pot connoisseur who lives near them and has journeyed to
Pakistan and Afghanistan to sample the best. Liz is also a doper,
and she's very short of money. She decides to grow some grass
for personal consumption, and she germinates some seeds she
finds in Tim's room.

Tim is Anne's fifteen-year-old son, who also smokes a lot
of pot. Anne disapproves of his smoking, but Tim says, "I can't
believe you don't want me to be honest about this, mum, that
you want me to lie." Anne doesn't see how she can stop him
smoking, but she doesn't like her son associating with dealers,
nor supplying his friends, which he has taken to doing. Kids
his age start coming to the door, and a camera and other things
go missing.

Liz gets a nice crop of seedlings. Then she finds Jay at the
market and asks for advice. Jay falls about laughing at the idea
of her seedlings. "That's pathetic! You can't use just any old
seeds, you'll have lousy pot. You want to grow sensi, and you
can only grow it from cuttings. Do you even have a place to
grow it? Maybe I should stop by."

That night, Jay drops in and Tim shows him around.

From the very beginning, Tim is a part of the plan. Tim's heavy smoking and dealing is one reason Anne starts growing grass: she wants to keep her son safe. She also wants to finance his college education.

Jay says their house is perfect. Under Jay's guidance, they fashion a special growing room in the attic. With the help of a carpenter, they lay down a floor, put up beams and plasterboard and place rubber sheeting on the floor. They install a big drum exhaust fan lined with charcoal to waft away the smell. They hang up lamps that stay on 16 hours a day and put silver foil on the walls to get maximum benefit from the lights. They install a new electrical circuit for the attic. They get large bins for the plants, which will be grown hydroponically, living on water and nutrients alone. Anne and Liz pay about £600 apiece for the set-up, and Tim helps with everything.

Jay gives them root cuttings from a mother plant. "Marijuana botany," says Anne, "attracts these really clever guys. That wonderful plant gave us years of great harvests." They grow eight, and only eight, plants because if they're caught with more they'll be considered providers, a much more serious offense than being users.

The beginning is easy, Anne says. "We have phenomenal growth! I run up the stairs twice a day just to see them grow. At first they're cute. Then they get big and demanding. They need feeding twice a day. You come out of the attic with the smell of skunk. But the worst chore by far is the flushing. When you grow grass hydroponically, in just rock wool and water, chemicals build up in the medium, which becomes toxic. So you have to flush out the plants' water every ten days. This means pouring five large watering cans of prepared water through the rock wool per plant. With eight plants, it takes at least three hours."

Flushing at Anne's involves a hose from the attic down to a sink on the top floor. One time when they have a houseguest, the hose comes loose, flooding the place and tripping the electricity. Their houseguest doesn't have an inkling about what's going on in the attic. Anne says, "I don't know what he thought about the flood."

At 12 weeks, the plants are ready for harvest. The harvesting and cleaning take the three of them five days, and after the harvest, there's the disposal problem. They have bags and bags of "jink"—stalks and big leaves of no commercial value. In the dead of night they drop their aromatic bags behind restaurants or in "skips" or dumpsters. "But with CCTV, it's always risky," Anne notes.

Jay is not only their adviser, he is also their buyer, which makes the whole operation quite safe. Jay wants only the buds, thick with resin. They give him bags of the stuff. That first harvest, she and Liz clear thousands of British pounds (Jay's fee is half of the first two harvests), and everyone is delighted. By the third harvest, Liz has moved out, they've amortized the equipment and Anne and Tim are making very good money. Then Jay becomes fussy and won't accept the less resinous buds. So they sell them to someone else. The whole thing is exciting, and Tim's college fund swells.

Anne's daughter, Jessica, 22, is not happy to learn about the attic farm. Worried about Anne getting caught, Jessica begs her to stop growing. "She was also alarmed at the appearance of our electrics—quite rightly," says Anne. "The operation relied upon water and electricity in close proximity. When I refused to stop growing, she got me a fire extinguisher and an escape ladder."

Although Jessica disapproves of the enterprise, cultivating marijuana creates a great rapport between Anne and Tim. "We bonded over growing," says Anne, who's divorced. "It made me a better mother. Tim had to develop responsibility, had to explore new areas, like building the growing room. He had to develop discretion, because he had to hide it from all of his friends—except his girlfriend. She helped with the harvest. None of his other friends knew about it, and none of mine did, either. And Tim stopped dealing. He didn't have to: he always had plenty of grass."

All told, Anne grows pot for about eight years, never getting caught. Jay visits now and then to sit with the plants and make suggestions. Anne gets interested in the growing equipment, and when she travels, she goes to industrial parks in other cities and countries to compare and contrast. She gets a lot of her own equipment from eBay, where there's a lively market in growing paraphernalia.

She herself never becomes a head. "I smoke half a joint to fall asleep. But though you sleep quickly, it's a light sleep."

"No other effects?" I ask incredulously. I feel a little sad for her.

She shakes her head. "I envy you so much, you get such pleasure from it, and it's so harmless."

"Well, I envy you being able to drink."

Anne stops growing her premium product when she asks her boyfriend Martin to move in. She feels she has to tell him about the attic, and when she does, he is adamant: she has to clear out the plants—a marijuana bust would be disastrous to his career. He offers to pay for Tim's supply, but they must clean out the attic. So Anne closes down operations, with some regret. "It's a lot of work and it's hard to do alone now that Tim's on his own." Tim has a good degree, a lucrative job in the City and a house in London he's bought with a friend. Anne continues, "But I miss the nurturing process. It's a great feeling, providing the plants with food, light, everything. You become mother nature!"

28
Quitting

Eight months after meeting Mark, I stop smoking pot. He neither smokes nor drinks; at our first dinner, when we lay out our liabilities (my age, 46, my three kids), he tells me he had a DUI (alone in his car, he hit a tree) and belongs to AA. He goes to several meetings a week. He's a young man: 30, blond, wholesome, smart. We have lots to talk about. He towers over me like a gentle giant. His skin is so tight over his muscles it feels like I'm stroking highly polished wood; he is so responsive that when I touch him he shivers. Although I hate driving at night and have claimed poor night vision for years, I now routinely get behind the wheel after dark so I can visit him at his place, 25 miles away. At least I-95 is well lit.

One time, I am "well lit" before Mark picks me up at home, and I feel distant, judgmental, self-conscious. That night, while I'm high, our effortless rapport is gone, and he seems awkward and naive. But when I come down, we are in our love cocoon again. Perhaps because we're so different in experience and background, we try to share each other's worlds as best we can. For some reason, I decide he likes country music, and I start listening to it for the first time. It's predictable but touching, and I tell him the song I like best. "That Was the River" by Colin Ray becomes our theme song. It takes months before we realize we're listening to the country music station just to please each other.

He takes recovery seriously and doesn't drink so much as a beer, so I never have a drink when I am with him, which is no special hardship. I know quitting pot will be harder, but I want to share his recovery mode with him. I'm no longer proud to be a pot-smoker but a little ashamed. And I could use a break. I've probably smoked every day since Jerome stopped nursing eight years ago. Stopping smoking is part of starting over, starting clean, and surely my breath will be better. Mark's breath is astonishingly sweet. He drinks a lot of Coca-Cola, and it may be bad for his teeth, but it's wonderful for his aroma. Sometimes, when he's sleeping, I adjust my breathing so I can inhale his breath, as if to absorb him. His skin smells sweet as well. I wish I could bottle it and dab it on when he's not around. Eau de Mark's Neck.

There's an additional reason I decide to stop smoking pot. My ex-husband is also with a partner who abstains, so he has quit smoking pot himself. We have always been competitive, and though our marriage is over, that dynamic lingers on. If Stan can quit, so can I.

I go to an open AA meeting with Mark in Norwalk. I'm impressed by the support they give each other and by how openly they talk about their lives. I see why meetings are important to him.

I don't have a ceremonial Last Joint. I'm low on grass, have only a little weak homegrown, but I don't throw it away. There's no drama about it: one day, I simply stop smoking. The next day I miss it, and I keep on missing it.

Finally, I go to a meeting in my village. I once noticed a group of dynamic and attractive people talking and smoking cigarettes outside the library. I asked a young woman, "What group is this?" expecting she would say a theater group. She hesitated before whispering, "AA."

I go to that meeting, relieved I don't see anyone I know. My problem isn't alcohol so it feels funny to introduce myself as an alcoholic, but this minor subterfuge seems the easiest way to proceed. There is no Narcotics Anonymous meeting near me, and people have said that NA is mainly for ex-heroin addicts, who might scoff at a mere dependence on pot.

The first night at AA I just listen. I'm not ready to tell my story; I just want to observe. I'm surprised at the number of people in the room who haven't had a drink for years or even decades. I wonder why they still come to meetings. Do they still need support or do they just crave intimacy? I leave with the Big Book, eager to start reading.

Now as the days go by, I feel very pleased with life, elated about my new purity. I feel a sense of possibility and joy and a great infusion of energy. I tell Mark about it on the phone.

"You're in the Pink Cloud," he says.

"The what?"

He explains that a few weeks after people stop drinking, they often have a period of bliss that might last a few days or weeks. The Pink Cloud always ends, but it's fun when you're in it.

I read the Big Book, trying not to worry about the Higher Power, as I have always been an atheist. I remind myself that AA has been very successful in getting people to stop drinking: why else would it be mandated after a DUI? I hope it will work well with me. I decide to stop worrying about the Higher Power and just get with the program. But after half a dozen meetings, I've had enough. Meetings keep reminding me that I've quit, and I don't want pot, or quitting pot, to be my focus.

Considering the centrality of weed in my life, I'm surprised, now, that I cannot recall if my marijuana fast lasted two years or three. I go to my journals to find out.

I've been keeping a journal since I was 11: sometimes avidly, sometimes not, in inverse proportion to my happiness. I write in cursive script in lined, spiral notebooks; now I'm on number 45. Sometimes I write once a month, sometimes, during periods of emotional turmoil, twice a day. Once I've finished a journal, I put it in an open plastic carton and never look at it again. The journals are important to me, though: that carton's in the front hall closet, ready to be hauled out if the house is on fire.

I go to that closet, remove the tennis bag and the exercise mat from on top of the carton and pull it out. The relevant volumes are numbers 32-35, which cover a three-year span. By contrast, my current volume, 44, covers a full two years and is only half-full. This reflects a present life of some equanimity; apparently, these days I'm only rarely compelled to communicate with myself to discover what I feel or to describe a stirring experience.

I take the old notebooks up to my study, stretch out on the striped couch and start reading volume 32. I soon see why I never bother rereading my journals. The pages are repetitive, inelegant and raw. I waste little time on niceties of description or style. And some of my preoccupations, especially concerning writing, fame and sex, haven't changed in 20 years. This in itself is depressing, reason enough to stop reading. But I do have a mission: to determine exactly how long I abstained and how I felt about it. Here are some unedited entries on the subject:

November 23, 1993

I have stopped smoking pot. It's hard. This is a habit I've had for 25 years, except during my pregnancies. But I want to be clean for Mark and for me. I'm tired of red eyes, low energy, morning coughing. I've been going to AA meetings to help kick. I now say, "I'm an alcoholic and an addict," which isn't entirely honest. And they value honesty so much! As do I. In this my new life I want to be straight.

It's the new me. I look the same but I listen to country music, love a much younger man, am compulsively honest and never get high.

(I just think about pot constantly and how I'm not smoking. I have it in the house but don't have papers!)

November 28, 1993

There are so many marijuana triggers for me. Eight days, and I'm very aware of how much a part of my life it was—and isn't. Another meeting, I guess. It's going to be hard to write without it—unless I remember that the last time I sought inspiration in a joint I fell asleep!

After every contact with Stan, I long to smoke dope to put it behind me.

December 11, 1993

Now I'm sitting on my sun-filled perch. Between nine and eleven it is a solarium at this time of year. I'd been avoiding it because I used to smoke pot here. But it is a wonderful place to sit.

December 23, 1993

An extraordinary development. My eyes have been aching and smarting every morning for weeks. This morning, with the pain worse than usual, I began to get indignant: is this the reward I get for giving up pot? Then I remembered that marijuana is sometimes given to glaucoma patients; it somehow helps relieve the pressure on the eye. It would be odd and ironic if I had to return to pot for medical reasons.

January 2, 1994

A New Year, a new me! Unmarried! Unaddicted! It's been six weeks since my last joint. It's been many months since I hoped for a return to marriage with Stan.

June 13, 1994

I'm getting stoned for the first time in six and a half months. I simply had this overwhelming desire to inhale, relax, tour my clean tidy house and be stoned in the hot tub. Andy just now came down: he'd smelled it in the upper garden and came running to the dell to say, "I caught you!" triumphantly. Shit. I'd suspected that smoking this joint would make me feel ashamed of myself—yet the urge was irresistible and the stuff was in the house—though not the papers. I used a Tampax wrapper, the traditional substitute.

June 15, 1994

So it was nice but not magical to be stoned again—but how fatigued I was after dinner! I'm not tempted to repeat the experiment, so in a way it's good I did it. Now I don't long for it at all. All that sneaking around!

July 14, 1994

Do I miss smoking pot? Once in a while. Yesterday I had such an unpleasant encounter with a client, a lawyer who set about "proving" his book was good, that I would certainly have gotten stoned if there had been fixings here. Instead I swam at the beach.

Dec 22, 1995

I've just smoked up the last of my homegrown from three years ago. It's been so mild it hasn't posed much of a temptation, and I've lived largely grass-free for about two years. Still tonight, I wanted to smoke, so now there's no grass in the house for the first time since I was married.

March 22, 1996

I'm thinking of buying some marijuana again. I think I can be an occasional smoker. At least, I hope so.

December 25, 1996

For the first time in years I'm going to buy dope. I've missed smoking pot, and I want to find a way to do it sensibly. If only there weren't this hiding and paranoia around it!

January 11, 1997

So I broke down and bought half an ounce of marijuana: my first dope buy in years. I always forget how fatigued pot makes me, and how paranoid. Still, of course it's a pleasure, and now when I'm alone in the house, as now, it will be a constant possibility, a pull toward the past. It's a return to my late, lamented freelance life.

January 17, 1997

In the eight days since buying the pot I've gotten stoned five times. This doesn't seem to be something I can do in moderation: it controls me, I'm afraid. Here I am in 12-degree weather on my perch with its windows and views, sucking in smoke because I'm alone and because I began reading an old Time *piece on pot and felt the need for it. Oh, any pretext will do now it's in the house. The restraints are kids, work, driving, looks, energy-drain. I must try to decide on a respectable level (twice a week) of pot use and stick to it. If I can.*

February 5, 1997

Whenever I smoke, Jerome knows—and jeers—even though I do it outdoors. He must smell it on my breath or clothes.

March 10, 1997

I can't smoke pot as casually as I used to. It's so fatiguing to me now. It takes a day to recover! I've lost the chemistry to tolerate the drug. To think I used to smoke two and three times a day!

April 27, 1997

And now I'm smoking dope just as much as before, with only a few caveats (Simon and Jerome must not be around; I must be outdoors; I can't drive or go to work afterwards). Back to twice a day.

After that, there's no mention of pot for months. So I stop reading. I've learned what I came to my journals for: I was basically smoke-free for about three years, though there were a couple of lapses. I also see that I can no more smoke sensibly than an alcoholic can have just one drink. If I'm smoking at all, I'm smoking every day, usually more than once. If I quit again, I'll probably have a few weeks of eye pain and a little more energy, but I won't be in some new, wonderful place. I'll simply be me, without weed—and that's a strange thought.

29
Bullhorn

It's a July evening, 1986, and Stan and I have just made a three-ounce buy at Ephraim's before leaving for the country. A long drive awaits, with Stan at the wheel and rock 'n roll on the radio. Before we leave the parking space outside Ephraim's, I roll us a joint from our new batch. This is our summer supply and I'm eager to taste it; so as we pull out, I light up.

I take a hit and pass it to Stan, who drives well on pot. We're at a red light on our way to the FDR. He passes the joint back to me. Suddenly, our car is floodlit: there's a spotlight on us. We hear a bullhorn: the voice, unbelievably, bellows, "Put out that joint!" Terrified, I snuff the joint into the ashtray and look up to see a police officer in an unmarked van in the right lane staring down at us. "Sorry, officer," I manage. He removes the spotlight and gives a disgusted, dismissive wave. The light turns green. He looks away, *and we each drive off.* He has places to go, better things to do than to bust us for pot. He turns a corner.

I lament my stupidity, lighting up in the car after making a buy, but we are giddy with relief. I suspect the evening would have ended differently if we'd been young and black.

30
Jamaica and Tortola

It's February, 1980, and we have just landed in Jamaica for a week's vacation with the kids, who are six and one. As soon as we step outside the airport we smell ganja, and as we walk to the car rental company with our children and suitcases, a young man offers us a baggie. We smile and shake our heads, for although we plan to buy some soon (bringing grass to Jamaica is like bringing coals to Newcastle), it doesn't seem smart to make a deal in the airport environs.

We drive our rental car toward our hotel on the other side of the island. Soon, the children are asleep in the back seat, and we are traveling through fields in the interior. At a stop sign by an intersection, two teenage boys wave us down and ask if we'd like to buy any pot. One produces a baggie, and the other names a price. Stan and I look at each other. Why not? We'll need to buy some soon, and the price is very good. Money and baggie are exchanged, and we continue on our way. I'm thinking that surely Jamaica is the pot-smokers' Jerusalem, the center of the culture, the spiritual source. Stan finds some rasta music on the radio and all is well as we roll merrily along.

Soon, the road curves to the right, and on the other side of the curve are two slender young men in uniform. One wears a cap. They signal our car to a stop and peer in. "Do you have any drugs?" asks the one with the cap.

"Drugs?" says Stan. "Of course not."

"You have drugs," he insists.

"We don't have drugs, we're on a family vacation."

"If you have any drugs," says the other, "you'd better tell us now, because we'll find them, and it will be worse for you."

"No drugs," says Stan.

Andy wakes up and looks on silently. The two guys who are questioning us are the only people in sight, and I begin to get nervous.

The guy without the cap puts his head into the driver's window and gives a sniff. "I think you have some drugs here," he says. He turns to me, and I can feel the blood leave my face. "Madam, please give me your drugs."

"I don't know what you're talking about," I tell him haughtily. (If the pot is found I plan to say, "It's not a drug, it's an herb.") My heart is thumping, but my voice is steady and a little outraged. "We're just tourists. We don't *have* any drugs."

Simon starts whimpering fretfully.

"We can search the car, you know," says the guy with the cap. But it seems more like a question than a threat.

"You won't find a thing," says Stan. "Now if you'll please back away, we need to get to our hotel." He puts the car in neutral and gives it some gas.

To our surprise, the young men move to the side of the

road. We drive on.

I look back. They are standing by the side of the road, no doubt ready for the next rental car.

"That was so weird," I say. "Just after we'd bought some."

"No coinkydink," says Stan. "It's a set-up. Their friends are down the road selling pot, and they think the tourists who buy it will be so frightened they'll bribe the 'police' to get off."

"I wonder if their uniforms are bogus."

"No tourist would know. So it's the perfect little scam."

"But scary!" I say. "Weren't you scared?"

"Petrified." Then we are laughing.

"I wonder if the dope's any good," I say.

"It smells good."

An hour or so later, we determine that even our scam-dope is fine. Excellent, in fact, and we have a fine time in Jamaica.

❉

In 1979, we take our first Caribbean vacation, to Tortola. We've brought our own pot along, rolled in joints, in a baggie in one of the baby's disposable diapers. To get to Tortola, we change planes in St. Thomas, which is where we go through customs. The customs officer is a tall and formidable figure who eyes us with suspicion. But there's just no way, I think, that he is going to search the diaper bag. He asks Stan to open his suitcase and rummages through it. He goes through Andy's backpack, which is stuffed with toys. He goes for the diaper bag and opens the zipper.

I feel my face turn white and the room start to spin. Boom, boom, boom: that must be my heart.

And now the officer puts his hand in the bag and starts feeling around.

Stan reaches for my arm to steady me.

The customs officer removes his hand and zips up the bag, seemingly disappointed. "You may go now."

I can scarcely move my legs. We move on through the terminal to our plane, which is tiny.

"We are *never* bringing dope across borders again," I tell Stan. He agrees. I have every intention of keeping that pledge.

Tortola is where we snorkel for the first time. We have rented a car called a "Gurgel," and Andy says over and over again, "I put the snorkels in the Gurgel." It's a very rough drive on a perilous, rutted road to get to the snorkel beach, which means most tourists stay away. We bounce along for 15 minutes, raising dust. Finally, the road spills onto a beach, with a guesthouse and restaurant to the right and white sand to the left. There are perhaps a dozen people on the beach.

Soon, we are putting on our masks and fins and walking backward into the warm Caribbean. Andy, who is six, takes to snorkeling at once and glides by my side easily. He's at that stage when he can swim underwater but hasn't learned to breathe, so the snorkel is perfect for him, as it's basically a tube you clamp in your mouth that curves above the water and into the air. I swim by his side, looking through the crystalline blue water at the sea floor. White sand. A little sea grass. A bleached piece of bone coral. Then I see a brain coral the size of a basketball.

It's a marker: a lazy breast stroke later, we are immersed in what seems like a teeming aquarium. Little blue and white striped fish nibble at pink and orange coral. A three-foot-long silvery fish approaches and is gone. Spiny sea urchins lurk beneath mahogany seaweed, and a clown fish hovers under an overhang. A ghostly angelfish drifts by. A hundred yellow fish the size of a child's hand waft near us. We are gripping each other and pointing.

When we finally stand up, our hands are wrinkled and our faces bear the marks of the diving masks. Snorkeling has left us speechless. We take off our fins and walk to shore. By the time we reach our towels, we are almost dry. Soon, I stay with Andy while Stan slips into the undergrowth to smoke a joint. Later, I will do the same, so the fish will be even more vibrant and vivid than before. And, indeed, pot adds an ecstatic dimension to the afternoon, as it so often does, until fatigue sets in.

It turns out that this is one of the best snorkel beaches in the world. In the years to come, I'm often disappointed by snorkeling. I'm annoyed that so often you need a boat to get to the reef, and regretful that the fish are never as various and colorful and plentiful as off that beach in Tortola long ago. So here's the question: is it really ideal to start at the top? An introduction to something at its best increases the chance you'll do it again, but doesn't it also set you up for disappointment ever after?

31
Six Toes

I have easy pregnancies: no morning sickness, no moodiness, no dark blotches, no stretch marks. I like how I look; it's nice to walk the streets of Manhattan, especially in summer, and not be considered sex bait. I like how strangers feel they can talk to me about babies just because I'm pregnant. It helps that my babies are actively wanted. It takes me a year to get pregnant with Andy, and, five years later, it takes me several months to get pregnant with Simon.

About a month before Simon is born, we move to 11th Street between Fifth and Sixth avenues in Greenwich Village. It's one of the most beautiful blocks in New York, and our apartment is one of the most eccentric. It's a walk-up on the third floor, with seven diminutive rooms accessed by a 34-foot-long hall. The miniature living room is a right-angle triangle, with a proboscis into the street and a working slate fireplace on the slanted side. Sliding doors lead to our tiny bedroom. Six of the rooms overlook a grimy airshaft, and there is exactly one closet and one bathroom in the entire apartment, off that long hallway. I read somewhere that a room can be listed as a bedroom only if it has a closet: otherwise, it must be called a den. So we are lodged in a 0-bedroom 4-den apartment.

No matter. I am now living across the street from my cousin Jackie; one block west of my dear friend Celia; one block north of my great friend Regina (with whom I will produce *Paul Bowles)* and a few blocks away from my oldest friend Jane, who lives in Westbeth. It feels like I'm on a university campus, with all my friends close by, but I'm in the middle of Greenwich Village, where I grew up. I feel a thrill of pride when I see tourists frowning over their maps. As a child of ten, I'd observe tourists and think: of course they want to be here, in the best neighborhood of the best city of the best country in the world! Now as an adult, when I get up at night, I play a little game. I go to the projecting portion of the living room and look out to Sixth Avenue. My game is how many seconds it takes until I see someone in the street. No matter what time I wake up, 3:30, 4:30, 5:00, it's never more than 30 seconds before there is someone out there, often walking toward the Korean fruit and vegetable store that never closes at all. This sense of activity going on around the clock always satisfies me, and I go back to bed happy.

Although I'm in my ninth month of pregnancy, I manage to settle us in and paint woodwork and put up curtains. My nesting instinct is ferocious. When I feel labor pains, Stan takes Andy across the street to stay with my cousin, then takes me to the hospital in a taxi. It is not a complicated birth, nor is it painless. And then there's that joyful reward. I hear, "It's a boy."

He's a dear little, dark-haired baby. Stan keeps counting his toes again and again, thinking he's seeing things. Then the doctor says, "Polydactylism. He has six toes." On each foot, his tiny pinky toe splits to a Y. The doctor says, "We can operate on him when he's two years old."

"Operate?" I ask. "Why?" It turns out there's no special reason, besides cosmetic. Six toes won't hamper his stride nor impair his health, and I'm thinking they're kind of cute. And they'll probably make him ineligible for the draft. This is the legacy of living through the Vietnam War.

I remember how Stan evaded the draft. He wanted to be declared 1-Y: unfit for psychiatric reasons. I suppose one would think twice about this strategy today, when such a designation might follow one around forever, impeding one's future career, but he wanted to avoid Vietnam at any cost. He pondered over how he could convince the draft board that they should reject him, and decided that rather than adopt a phony madman persona, he would merely exaggerate certain aspects of his personality. He prepared for the induction by taking LSD and staying up all night. He was just coming down, clammy and hollow-eyed, pupils still dilated, when he changed for the draft board. He wore his oldest clothes: a tattered green army jacket, old jeans and a reeking T-shirt. He hadn't shaved for a week, at a time when stubble was for bums, not metrosexuals. He looked a mess, but he had his wits about him. After passing the physical, he gamed the questionnaire and was sent to the psychologist, who asked him some questions. Most of the time, Stan was silent and utterly unresponsive, but when the psychologist asked, for the third time, "Do you know why you're here?" Stan suddenly screamed, "No, I don't!"—terrifying the doctor, who sent him out of the room in a hurry. Stan got his 1-Y.

So when I first see Simon's feet, my first thought is: it's the perfect draft deferment. All he has to do when called up is to say he needs custom-made boots because of his toes…But my second thought is: am I to blame? Polydactylism—having more than five digits on a hand or foot—doesn't run in my family, nor Stan's. I worry that perhaps the pot I smoked before I knew I was pregnant (we had some strong stuff one night with a Hollywood producer) somehow produced a mutation that gave Simon those toes. And it's not just the toes I'm concerned about. Now the doctor is telling me that sometimes polydactylism is associated with "anomalies" in the organs. He takes Simon away to be tested. I am left in terror. What if my baby has something wrong with his kidneys, his stomach, his heart? How will I ever forgive myself? The hour that I should be exultant I am petrified.

The doctor returns with magnificent news. Simon's organs are fine; he's in perfect health. So I try to ease up on myself. After all, I didn't know I was pregnant when I had that joint at that party, and, besides, there's absolutely no evidence that marijuana is teratogenic—causing malfunctions in the fetus. Nor is there a link between cannabis and polydactylism. I tell myself if there was such a link, half the children in Jamaica would have six toes.

I fly the marijuana flag, yet perhaps on some deep level I

think it's bad to smoke weed and that I should be punished, because a certain guilt about those toes remains to this day. And to this day, I'm happy that we didn't have today's technologies when I was pregnant with Simon. Our current ultrasound images are clear enough so that Simon's toes would have been counted and noted. I might have been warned that these toes often accompany organ "anomalies" with life-changing consequences. I might have been told that the baby could be severely disabled or in chronic pain. I might have wanted to terminate the pregnancy. No Simon in the world? This is such a terrible thought I feel the blood in my arms go cold, and I'm profoundly grateful for the fuzzy ultrasound images of the late seventies.

When Simon is three months old, I take him to baby swim classes. I have a hunch that his extra toe might give him an advantage in swimming, so why not start him early? The water is warm, and the mothers are taught to blow air into their babies' faces so they won't inhale, and then plunge them through the water. The babies look ecstatic, the mothers are thrilled and the pool must be the happiest place in New York.

Simon never becomes a competitive swimmer, nor does he ever need a draft exemption, but he always makes beautiful footprints in the sand.

32
High at Home

The year is 1970, Stan and I are newlyweds and everyone we know smokes pot. We keep ours in a white, three-inch-high Limoges porcelain canister with the word "Marijuana" centered upon it in Old English Text. This little canister sits on our mantelpiece. Guests invariably lift up the top, look inside and take a sniff. Zig-Zag Wheat Straw rolling papers and matches from Max's Kansas City, our local restaurant, are at the ready in a green glass box nearby. At Max's, the steak special is $4.95.

We live in a rent-controlled apartment on East 24th Street. The neighborhood is sooty and industrial, and the bedroom gives onto an airshaft so dingy we never open the curtains. There are hookers on the corner, and once there was a shoot-out right outside our windows. But the space is nice, with a large living room, a fireplace and a kitchen with French windows overlooking Miller's Saddle Shop. We pay $160 a month, and even then, it's a steal.

The apartment reeks of marijuana, which seems like a good smell to me. It lurks in the folds of the curtains, in the cushions of the couch, in the nap of the rugs. It greets us as we open the front door. Sometimes, in summer, we return to a blast of cold marijuana air. Con Edison offers lower rates the more energy you use, so we often leave the air conditioner on for seven or eight hours, just for the delightful shock of the cold upon returning from the steaming summer streets.

Often the first thing we do upon coming home is to head for the porcelain canister. Stan usually rolls the joints: he's better at it than I am, more mechanical in general, whereas I excel at the abstract. I am writing a dissertation on "Person and Persona: Narrative Voice in John Updike's Fiction." Stan started out as a cameraman, but has now found steady work as a film editor. He is more visual; I am more verbal. We have neatly divided the talents between us, I feel, and I'm sure that we'll always be together. We are in our twenties and very affectionate physically. I feel sorry for all the couples who no longer hold hands.

Pot agrees with both me and Stan. It feels like a happiness potion, and it enhances most of the things we like to do. Our lives are soaked in the stuff: it is woven into the fabric of our domesticity. After a day in the editing room (sometimes smoking with the director), Stan always rolls a jay before dinner. He can be rather saturnine, but as soon as he gets high, he makes some pleasant and appreciative remark. Perhaps he likes the song that's playing on WNEW, the first "album" radio rock station in New York. Perhaps he has something nice to say about how dinner smells. Perhaps he notices what I'm wearing.

Do I discount all this because he's high? Not at all. I'm high, too, of course.

I serve the meal. We eat a full dinner at home most of the time, and it is the highlight of our day. Stan is devoted to food, and he always offers a measured critique of the meal. He says, "It could use a little more thyme. Other than that, it's very good." When you're high you're more appreciative of food, more sensitive to its nuances. We wouldn't dream of going to a restaurant without getting stoned.

When we eat in, we rarely have dessert, though, once in a while, we will have "candy bar," which Stan has invented. This is a deconstructed candy bar—with deluxe ingredients. When we have guests, we sometimes set out little bowls of dark chocolate, almonds, raisins, and coconut. It's the perfect answer to the marijuana munchies.

At around this time, I have my first bout of what I will later come to call "restaurantitus." We are at some Greenwich Village restaurant and have eaten a big meal, savoring every mouthful and tasting everything on each other's plates, even the garnishes. We order dessert, and I finish every last scrap of my crème brûlée, even though I'm bursting. Stan pays the check, and we stand up to leave. Suddenly, all the colors leach from the room and I see only black and gray. I am dizzy and swaying. "Are you all right?" Stan asks, and I shake my head, gasping, "I have to get out, I need air." Now I can scarcely see anything at all, and he guides me outside and into the cold night. Finally, we reach the sidewalk, and I lower myself down. I am nauseated. I am having a blackout. I want to lie flat on the sidewalk, but Stan holds me up, and I put my head between my knees. Cars rush by in front of me, people stroll along in back of me. I am glad I am not a celebrity, and I can faint, or die, without attracting attention. It takes 20 minutes before I'm strong enough to stand up and get into a taxi.

This episode frightens both me and Stan, yet over the next few years, it is repeated several times. The elements are always the same. I'm stoned. I've eaten a lot. Maybe I've had a glass of wine. And then I have dessert. I deduce that somehow pot must affect sugar metabolism, yet from one time to the next, Stan and I seem to forget where marijuana, rich food and dessert can lead me. Flat out on the floor of the ladies room—or on the sidewalk like some junkie.

Stan and I have a traditional marriage: he earns most of the money, and I do most of the housework. Nonetheless, I have elected not to change my name to his, which makes me "Ms. Hiller." As a title, "Ms." is brand-new and faintly ridiculous, but I see no reason to announce my marital status one way or another every time I give my name.

The Women's Liberation Movement is gaining momentum, and I go to a few consciousness-raising meetings. I share the feminist indignation about the lack of equal opportunity and equal pay for women. Until very recently, the newspaper "Help Wanted" is divided: jobs for men and jobs for women. Most of the good jobs are for men; women are basically restricted to being secretaries, nurses or teachers. This is the world I grow up in. As a girl, I always run my finger through newspaper lists of honors or awards, hoping to find a woman's name, but it almost never happens.

I subscribe to *Ms.*, the first women's magazine I've seen

with moral and political weight. Still, I never become part of an ongoing women's group. I'm content to assume the traditional role in my marriage, and I'm satisfied with my personal life. I don't fit in with most of the women at the groups; I am not sufficiently embittered. And many of the women seem frumpy, joyless, angry. I wouldn't want them for my friends. I wouldn't want to get high with them. If I like somebody, I want to get stoned with him or her so we can both feel good together in a similar way. I wish that the feminist movement would somehow embrace psychedelics, or at least pot, but I know this is unlikely.

I am quite sure that in 30 years or so—by the year 2000—marijuana will be fully legal in every state. Rumor has it that already R.J. Reynolds has registered Acapulco Gold as a brand name. I am confident that by the millennium there will be a pot-smoking car beside the bar car on commuter trains to the suburbs. I wonder whether that will significantly matter.

By 1972, I have received my doctorate, and I am temporarily "filling a line" at Brooklyn College. I'm teaching three different classes, and it takes me 60 hours a week to read and prepare and correct papers. Fortunately, we are able to save all the money I make. In May, I am told that the English Department cannot offer me a full-time position in the fall, only adjunct work. As this is a step down, and I am haughty in my youth, I spurn it, though I agree to teach two final courses in the summer. One of them is under-enrolled, so it is canceled. In the other, I have my students read *Lolita*. Since nothing is at stake, I don't work very hard, and I'm a much better teacher. I enjoy myself. I have no idea that I will never again teach full time at a college. There are simply no jobs in New York or Los Angeles, the only places where my husband's career can thrive.

In August, I get a check for the course I taught and a check for the course that was canceled. I immediately bank the first and cash the second. I lay out the extra money— $1500—in piles of twenties on the glass coffee table. When Stan comes home I declare, "They overpaid me! Look at that!" We do a little jig around the room.

I never think of returning the money; I figure this is severance pay. I'm bitter that Brooklyn College hasn't kept me on, since I graduated from there with honors, earned my PhD at Brown and thought they'd be glad to have me come back as a full-time faculty member.

My extra illicit money becomes part of the down payment we now have so we can look for a country house. Like many of our cohorts, we want to get "back to the land"—at least on weekends—never mind that our forebears were all urban Jews. As we search increasingly northward for something we can afford, we tell realtors that privacy is paramount. Basically, we don't want people seeing us smoke pot. We are, after all, doing something illegal, and there is still the sense that marijuana is for hippie liberals. We don't want to outrage the local rednecks (who will all be smoking dope themselves in another few years).

After several months during which we bid unsuccessfully on an old radio station in the Poconos and 15 acres of raw land near Woodstock, we find a small 1840s farmhouse in Delaware

County. From inside, you can't see any other houses, only trees and mountains. Stan smokes by the fireplace and by the stream and on the porch. I do not smoke. I am pregnant with Andy, my first. If my calculations are correct, he was conceived on our first night in our country house, on a foam mattress on the floor.

During my pregnancy, I give up marijuana and the three daily cigarettes I've permitted myself in the past. I find that I crave cigarettes more than I crave pot. I miss the smoke in my throat and in my lungs more than the high in my head. Yet after the baby is born, I never go back to cigarettes, while I do go back to marijuana—as fast as I possibly can.

Because pot is for celebration, a few hours after Andy is born, I hobble off to a stairwell and smoke a joint. Then how even more thrillingly happy I am that the baby is healthy and that the birth went well! Back in the dim room with him, I bring the baby to my shoulder and put my nose to his head. I am feeling postpartum euphoria, which will persist for several months.

I smoke pot very rarely while I'm a nursing mother, but out of nostalgia and habit, I continue to clean it. Some people object to the strainer method of cleaning grass and say that the resin gets scraped off by the mesh, but that seems far-fetched to me, and the final result is easy to roll and gets us high fine.

So on this summer's day, alone with the baby in the farmhouse, I'm about to start cleaning some grass when Andy, who's three months old, awakens. I put the bowl with the strainer and the pot on the kitchen table and race upstairs to get him. I bring him down with me to the kitchen table, which is by the back door and next to a picture window overlooking a small meadow. I start nursing the baby. I see someone turning the corner of the house and approaching, coming to the back door, and I hunch over myself and the baby for modesty.

It's Howie, a houseguest of our neighbor's, and I tell him to come in. Andy goes on chomping at the breast, and Howie enters and starts brightly asking if he can make a phone call as my neighbor's line is out. Suddenly, he takes in the scene: me on the chair, half naked, nursing the baby, and the pile of brownish leaves in the strainer. His face changes. I don't know what shocks him more: the bare breast, the weed or the possible combination: am I smoking while nursing? Howie, at 45, is in a different generation from mine, and he's now rendered speechless. I direct him to the phone upstairs and he races from the kitchen, escaping my depravity. I feel like a degenerate. At times like these, my commitment to cannabis falters. Am I doing something wicked?

I resume regular pot-smoking when I stop nursing. I'd probably smoke more if it didn't make me so sleepy. The better the pot, the more it fatigues me. Some will claim that not all pot is fatiguing, but I've found a high correlation between certain physical symptoms and potency. If it's good, it makes my mouth very dry, it gets my eyes very red and, after an hour or two, it makes me very sleepy.

Rumor has it that Jack Nicholson smokes all the time and that he once took a four-hour break and considered it a marijuana fast. By comparison, my own smoking doesn't seem excessive.

My parents know I smoke, but not how much. In the dubious belief that the people I love will enjoy what I enjoy, I want to share my drug of choice with the three of them: my father, my mother and my stepfather, Antoine, who is no longer married to my mother.

My father is the first to try. He gave up smoking cigarettes the day when the Surgeon General's report came out in 1964, which gives him the most smoking experience of the three. So I don't have to teach him how to inhale. And he's game, but not eager, for the experience. As a Marxist and an American Communist, he doesn't have much interest in the pleasure drugs provide, but he also wants to be close to me and understand my generation. So late one summer's afternoon in the country, we share a joint. "Hold it in as long as you can," I tell him. And he's good at that, but the pot doesn't seem to affect him very much. He says "wow" at the sunset sky, but he's been incongruously using that expression for several months now. Then he stretches out on the sofa and takes a long nap.

After that, if I'm smoking, I usually offer him some, and he usually declines. Apparently, I haven't made a head out of him. He's not much of a drinker, either. He is busy organizing, volunteering, going to meetings.

My mother's a better candidate for marijuana, I decide, because she's more of a hedonist, more of a sensualist. She values the present moment and is always open to new experience. We sit in the living room and I pass her the joint. She fills her mouth with smoke then tips her head back, expecting that gravity will send it down her throat. "You have to breathe it in," I say, and she breathes it in and has a coughing fit. I run to get her a glass of water. After a while, we start again. She draws on the joint and I tell her, "Now bring some nice, fresh, cool air into your mouth and breathe it all into your lungs." She inhales—coughs and splutters.

We try twice more before she succeeds. "I think I feel it already," she says hopefully. "I think I'm potted already."

I say, "You can't possibly feel it from that. Take some more." It's the same ordeal all over again. She finally manages to ingest three or four tokes, after which she gets animated and chatty. But she is always animated and chatty. Do I expect some magical "new mother" to emerge? Do I think our good rapport will become even better? Do I think she will suddenly start loving The Who? If so, I'm disappointed. And once again, I have failed to make a marijuana convert.

I have high hopes for my stepfather, Antoine, because of our red pill conversations. When I am ten, long before Prozac, he asks: "If a red pill could make people happy, would you take it?" He always avers that he would, while my mother gets indignant at the idea.

Now that I have found my own "red pill," I expect my stepdad to exult and enjoy it with me. But he will have none of it. "I hate every form of smoking," he says. "I hate the way it feels. I hate what it does to my throat. And I hate what it does to the breath. I could never go out with a woman who smokes anything. It's too bad you've developed this horrible habit."

"But it feels so good," I protest. "And the red pill! You wanted everyone to take the red pill!"

He brushes off this allusion. "First of all," he says, "marijuana's illegal. You could go to jail."

"Highly unlikely for a first offense."

"And second of all, it's very dangerous."

"Pot? Dangerous? There hasn't ever been an overdose in all of human history. Smoke too much and you just go to sleep."

"That's not true," he says. "Pot can make you go insane. When I was growing up in Cuba, there were certain mental hospitals that were just for the *marihuaneros*. People who'd gone crazy from smoking too much."

"That sounds highly dubious," I tell him—but what do I really know? "It's just something they said to scare the children."

"It's the truth," he assures me. "I wouldn't touch it if you paid me."

So my dreams of getting high with Antoine go up in smoke.

I light a joint with my husband and lament how ineffective I am as a proselytizer.

"Maybe it's a generational thing," he suggests.

"A mindset," I say. "You have to have a certain willingness, the right preparation, even the right vocabulary."

"Vocabulary?"

"Look—in the nineteenth century, all these women were taking these 'ladies' medicines,' which were really laudanum or morphine. Yet you never read about any of them getting high! They didn't have the word for it and so they never felt it."

"I suppose as a writer you feel if it can't be expressed it isn't really real?"

"Something like that," I admit. "But what's 'real,' anyway, about a mental condition or a mood?"

"Beats me," says my husband. "Is that thing in your hand still lit?"

33
Updike's Protégée

I take my orals on my dissertation with a hand-rolled cigarette alight. There's only tobacco inside, but I'm hoping my supervisors will be taken off-guard. Why do I have this constant need to shock? Because as a child I was such a good little girl, often compared to an angel? Or is my identification with my generation so strong I must constantly proclaim it?

I have written my dissertation on John Updike, who is only 39 years old when I start my close reading of his oeuvre. At this point, he's published dozens of short stories, much light verse, a lyrical novel about an old-age home, a myth-like novel based on his father's life and, of course, the scandalous *Rabbit Run*, still his most recognized achievement. I am drawn by the grace of his prose and the stinging precision of his descriptions. His sexual frankness is another attraction: erotic candor through a literary sensibility. In later years, he wins a lifetime Bad Sex Writing award, which seems unfair, though I hear he takes it with good grace. We should distinguish between bad sex writing and writing about bad sex, the latter of which Updike does better than anyone. (Good sex, naturally, is harder to write about.)

As far as I know, mine is among the first dissertations on his work: the first is "Pastoralism and Anti-Pastoralism in John Updike's Fiction," which I abbreviate in my notes to "Pasta and Anti-Pasta." Sitting in the main branch of the New York Public Library or at the graduate school library at CUNY, I write, in longhand, my doctoral thesis. When it's all typed up, it's 350 pages, and my friend Jane reads it all. She endears herself forever to me when she says, "I wish it were longer."

My doctoral committee wants to know if I've met Updike, and they are more impressed when I tell them I have than by the subtle narrative strategies I discuss in detail in my dissertation. I explain to the professors that I spent a day in Ipswich with him, and they want to know all about him. Why did he grant me the interview, they ask, for Updike is said to deny these requests. I explain that I am writing an article, "Updike at Forty," on spec for the *New York Times Magazine*.

When we meet, Updike asks how old I am. "Twenty-five," I tell him.

"My goodness, that's young, and how did you persuade the *Times* to let you come interview me?"

Is there a tiny flirt in there? I hope so, although my husband, Stan, is very much in evidence, taking black and white photographs. The flirt, if such it is, will never go further than this, and in a way it's mere courtesy. At the time it's polite to flirt mildly with a young woman. I also recognize in Updike the competitiveness of one smart young person for another—

although his achievements by age 25 (poems and stories in *The New Yorker*, a prize-winning first novel) far surpass mine. I only have the PhD.

I explain about the dissertation and how I've been scrutinizing his fiction for two years. I turn on the tape recorder, and our interview begins. I have written three pages of questions, but I don't need to ask them. He talks gracefully hour after hour at the smallest prompt. We start in his house and move on to his office in town. Stan takes a great picture of me bending over my clipboard, long, wavy hair over my shoulders, a smile on my lips. Updike is in profile on the other side of the frame. I am interviewing my literary hero and loving it.

His best line of the day? Five words: "Prose can always be better" —a phrase I remember every day I write

I turn in a gracious, 20-page profile, "Updike at 40." I am too much in awe of my subject to write a piece with much edge, but I think it's well-informed. I send the piece to him so he can approve his quotes. He writes back, "The quotes all seem fine—some of them, indeed, much better and funnier than anything I could have said. My reservation about the piece is that there is, in the first ten pages, too much about me as a sweetie-pie and community drone, and not enough about the writing…this impression gets a bit altered in the second half, but by this time you've gotten us pretty thoroughly bored with this guy…As is, I don't think it's sexy (in a non-sexy sense) enough to make it in the Times, between those articles on Inside the ARVN and The Pill-Twenty Years After."

He proves prophetic. The *Times* vote is 3-2 against, and

while *Esquire* is initially interested, they ask me to cut it in half and I remove only two pages—I can't bear to lose anything! So they turn it down, too.

Stan and I go to Europe for a couple of months, for a much belated honeymoon. I nonchalantly miss the doctoral ceremony at Brown, something I will later regret, though at the time, formalities like this are scorned by all our friends. I return home and upon my return, I tuck away "Updike at 40" and go on to other projects.

I am not, at the time, career-oriented, but now I see that if the article had been taken by the *Times* or *Esquire* or another respected publication, it might have made a difference in my professional life. I might have done more journalism, I might have become better known. I might even have gotten a full-time college teaching job (where, in the politically correct decades that followed, I would have been absolutely miserable).

Alas, Updike makes Erica Jong's career, not mine, with his ecstatic review of *Fear of Flying*, a perfect match of book and reviewer. (The book's gusto is enough like mine so that Anne asks in a letter if I wrote *Fear of Flying* under a pseudonym.)

When *Rabbit Redux* is published, I am pleased to find marijuana is a major element in the book. During my interview with him (of course I have to ask him about pot), he says grass doesn't agree with him and makes him tired the next day. Apparently, by *Rabbit Redux*, his body has adjusted, and every time one of his characters lights up, I do, too.

As the years and decades go by, I send Updike one novel manuscript after another, reminding him of my precocious interest in his work and hoping for a blurb. I never hear back.

In the nineties, my agent has the idea of putting all of my sexy short stories into one book. I have to juice up a few, which process proves highly enjoyable. *Skin: Sensual Tales* makes the rounds for three years before being taken by Carroll & Graf.

As always, I send Updike the manuscript. Two weeks later, I come home from work at lunchtime to find that the mail's come early, and there's a small typed envelope . . . from Him. The letter reads, "You could say I said: Catherine Hiller writes with a fine directness and clarity . . . Good luck with your book, and your good, brave and joyful writing."

I am on air. It is a father's hug, a teacher's A++, a lifetime validation and reward.

The publisher puts the quote above the title, but the book gets few reviews and has tepid sales. Still, I always like giving people the book because of that quote on the cover.

Things continue to get worse in the publishing business, as in my own career. One day in 2008, I Google myself for the first time, and on page three I come across a six-month-old article in the *London Times* in which I am described as "Updike's protégée." I stare at it, horrified. Since my interview in Ipswich with him, I have seen Updike only two or three times, always at public readings, at which I linger at the end to have a few words with him. What if Updike finds out and thinks I gave the *Times* this misinformation? I am tempted to write a letter to the *London Times* denying this mischaracterization, but I figure it will only stir up the issue again. Best to let it just go away.

I feel saddened and ashamed because I can't help thinking how glorious it would have been if I had been Updike's protégée!

34
Wedding

Stan and I plan to marry on the winter solstice, 1969. In September, I find a white linen croquet dress from the 1890s hanging in an antique store window, with the sun shining on it so it glows. It has eyelet embroidery and 20 fabric-covered buttons running down the back. Mesmerized, I walk into the store and into the dressing room. The dress fits as if made to my form, and I buy it, even though $125 seems very expensive for an old dress.

Dress secured, I immediately become more enthusiastic about planning the wedding. We don't want a conventional wedding; we want a celebration that reflects who we are. As it turns out, in our attempt to be our hippie selves yet honor the wedding traditions, the dress is our only unqualified success.

We decide against engraved invitations: we hire a calligrapher instead. We find one by calling Everything for Everyone, an organization matching seekers and providers. The invitations are beautiful, and I like Miriam, the calligrapher, so much I invite her to the wedding, but the ink on the envelopes smears when wet, and one invitation can't be delivered and is sent back. For reasons now opaque, I write my thank-you notes on origami paper. I never see Miriam again, except in the wedding photos.

We don't want anything as conventional as a traditional wedding album, with artificial groupings of people and posed moments—wife feeds a forkful of cake to her husband, they both look thoughtfully at her hand with its new ring, etc. No, Stan wants our wedding to be documented, rather than conventionally photographed, so he hires a documentary photographer and has him shoot mainly candid shots, all black and white. The results are certainly original. The photographer might have been reporting on anomie in America: there's my jolly paternal grandmother on a chair looking deeply alone; there's our glamorous friend Robin staring disconsolately out at the Long Island Sound; there's a waiter on a break, leaning against a wall, smoking a cigarette. The photographer has taken our wedding and turned it into an Antonioni event. At least we have Froggy's pictures, I think.

Froggy is Stan's friend from NYU Film School, recently married himself. He's promised to take color photos to supplement the black and white ones, and I'm eager to see if there's a single shot of me and Stan in the same picture, smiling, something the official photographer has not managed to capture. After a couple of weeks, I ask Stan about Froggy's pictures. "He was tripping on mescaline," says Stan. "He forgot to load the film."

The music is about as successful as the photography. The

last thing we want is a *wedding band,* with its syrupy renditions of traditional songs and a corny bandleader pattering on. We're too sophisticated for any of that, so Stan hires a jazz band better known for its studio work than for its live performances. It does not burst into a scat version of "Here Comes the Bride" when I walk down the aisle, but plays something else entirely. They are cool, and they inspire a similar coolness in our guests. When it comes time to dance, few take to the floor, for the beat is subtle and elusive. When the band takes a break, we put on some Arabic music, and suddenly all the women on my side of the family—Syrian Jews—get up and begin moving their arms and their hips. Belly-dancing is part of our tradition. A few men join them, wielding napkins. The photos of these happy moments look strangely menacing.

Our final mistake is getting our friends high. We have a designated smoking room at the yacht club where we get married, and after the vows, our friends all troop into the room. We smoke joints we have rubber-stamped "Stan & Cathy." (Other contemporary weddings have cigarettes at each table with the name of the couple imprinted on them; we're just taking the idea one step further.) The pot is good, and after we go back to party, we become quiet and observant. While our parents' friends are drinking and getting ever jollier, our own set is zonked, introverted and fatigued.

Perhaps the photographs convey a certain truth, after all.

Luckily, the marriage is much more successful than the wedding, at least for the first 20 years.

35
Woodstock

It's 1969, and by August I'm getting anxious. For weeks, I've heard about a music festival in Woodstock, New York, with an incredible lineup of talent. The Jefferson Airplane! The Who! Jimi Hendrix! Janis Joplin! The Band! I think we should buy weekend tickets even though they're $35 each, but Stan has heard that they might be making a film of the festival, and maybe they will need him to shoot, and maybe we'll get to go free. This is too many maybes for me, and as the days pass, I grow increasingly irritable. I want to be at this gathering. What I revere about the counter-culture is the music: songs that inspire me to protest and dance, music that is relevant and inventive and radically different from the love-sick laments of the past. And here comes the greatest lineup of musicians ever, and I'm going to miss them, just because Stan won't commit.

Only days before the festival, Warner Brothers puts $25,000 into the production, and Michael Wadleigh, known in downtown New York as a brilliant cinematographer, is hired to direct the documentary *Woodstock*. The call goes out for people with 16 mm cameras to help shoot. This includes Stan. Everybody is very excited. With any luck, we think, this film can be as good as *Monterey Pop*, and rumor has it that Bob Dylan himself may appear.

We arrive in Bethel, New York, on Thursday afternoon. On the highway, we see cars full of hippies going in the same direction we are, smiling and flashing the peace sign. We leave the highway and drive along the smaller road to the festival. At Brown, there are some hippies, or people who look like hippies: perhaps five percent of the student population. But everyone here is a flower child: thousands of boys and girls with long hair and dilated pupils who have arrived early and set up camp.

Stan takes some footage of kids dancing and smoking pot, and at night, we leave the festival site and return to the motel. The film crew does not camp in the mud: we sleep in dry rooms on clean sheets, and every morning, I set up the ironing board and iron my hair. It's very important to have straight hair, although the iron sometimes leaves burn marks on my arms.

On Friday, the crowd grows large, and by Saturday, it is dense and immense: a vast field of young people wearing jeans and T-shirts, beads and fringes, beards and bandanas. So many freaks! Woodstock is the coming-out party of my generation.

Stan is assigned to a platform to one side of the main stage, high up on a tower. Each major performer will be covered by three main cameras close to the stage and several cameras from other angles. We don't have the traditional slate or clapboard, so Stan writes the name of the group on a sheet of paper and shoots me holding it up. I display his scrawled sign for Santana.

It's astonishing how much good music there is, and how well it sounds whether you're near or far. The performers may look like dots, but you can hear the lead guitar dueling against the bass from a quarter of a mile away. When I'm not on the platform helping Stan or simply watching the concert, agog, I am mostly under the stage with the other girlfriends and assistants, changing magazines, which hold the film. Each reel of 16 mm film lasts 11 minutes, and when it's finished, it has to be changed, by feel, in a dark bag, with the exposed film placed in a can and the new film threaded into the magazine. Someone teaches me the technique, and I sit with the blackout bag and camera on my lap, like the others who are doing this. They look dreamy and abstracted as their hands work within the bags on their laps, as if they're masturbating.

I hear that all the Woodstock security guards are tripping. This does not strike me as entirely good news, but it makes me feel better about smoking pot on the platform.

It begins to rain again and a sickening smell emerges from the mud, with notes of cow shit and vomit. But everybody is lighthearted in the rain. We are here on a hillside making history! Chip Monk, the mellifluous MC, tells us we've closed down the New York Thruway! He tells us not to eat the brown acid—not because it's illegal, but because it's a bummer. He announces Joan Baez, and there she is, below us, Lady Madonna, with that voice like clear water over stones. Bob Dylan does not join her onstage (nor at the festival), but Crosby, Stills and Nash, whose first album has just come out and whose every song I know by heart, come to the stage and announce that this is their second public performance and they are "scared shitless!"

Shitless! I love the brute honesty and profanity! I love that the performers and stage hands and audience are all wearing the same clothes: old denim, soft cotton. I love the feeling of convergence: people with the same politics and outrage and values all gathered together. "Give me an 'F,'" says Country Joe (of the Fish), and we shout it back to him as helicopters fly above us. We are viscerally united in our politics and our passions. We are half a million people for each other.

American Cinematographer takes a picture of me and Stan on the platform. Stan, with his camera, looks focused and stern; I look enraptured It's a fine shot, and with that photograph, I finally make it to Stan's cork wall.

Stan goes on to become one of the editors of *Woodstock*. An earlier version of Santana's performance, edited by Martin Scorsese, begins with me holding up that piece of paper we used as an improvised clapboard, but when Stan is asked to re-cut the sequence, this opening does not jibe with his vision so he removes it. At the time, I am proud of him: the aesthetic has trumped the personal.

Now, all these years (and one divorce) later, I'm no longer happy that he cut me out of *Woodstock,* the movie that chronicles my generation's pivotal event. It would have been a cute beginning to the sequence, and I would have had two seconds on screen: young, grinning, straight hair flying in the wind.

36
Twenty

Stan and I meet at a party in Manhattan to which neither of us is invited. Indeed, we do not even know the host: we've each come with a friend. I am 20, a senior at Brooklyn College; Stan is 25, studying film at NYU. We are sitting on a sofa. I don't remember what we first chat about, but soon he starts telling me jokes from the *Two Thousand Year Old Man* LP by Mel Brooks, whom I haven't heard of. I start smiling.

A recent study has determined that women value a sense of humor in a man more than any other trait. I'm not surprised. A man who likes to laugh, and make you laugh, is probably not angry or self-important, and if you laugh at the same things, you probably share the same frame of reference and even hold the same values. In addition, I think laughter is in some sense surrender, and perhaps, unconsciously, women may associate one sort of surrender with another.

Stan makes me laugh a lot that night. When he goes off to get more chips, some cute guy asks me to dance. I love to dance, but I shake my head. I know if I get on the floor I might never talk to Stan again, that's just how parties are. So I wait on the sofa for Stan. That night, he drives me home to Brooklyn in his very tiny car: I've never been inside a Mini Cooper before. Stan tells me he worked on *Chafed Elbows,* an underground film I have heard of. I'm impressed. The next day, I fly to Berkeley to see Celia, and throughout my visit, I think about Stan and wonder if he smokes pot.

As it turns out, he does, and often. It's one of our many bonds. Sometimes we don't go out, we just go to his apartment, where we get high, clamp on pairs of headphones and listen to a new record album. The music pours into our heads. I accept this routine unquestioningly, never mentioning that it might be nice to talk while we listen or that music also sounds good on his speakers. The headphones, of course, keep us apart. He keeps his distance, which makes him maddeningly desirable. When he asks questions, it sometimes feels like he's interviewing me for a job rather than starting a conversation. Then he'll say something funny and I have to laugh.

Stan has a cork wall in his apartment on which are pinned black and white photographs: portraits of good-looking women; street scenes at night; rain beading on windshields; bare manikins in a store window. Photography is his hobby, and my ambition is to get myself up on the cork.

I graduate from Brooklyn College *summa cum laude.* There are nine of us *summas* in a class of 1700. Marijuana hasn't harmed my concentration nor fuzzed my memory, and I'm offered a full fellowship to study English in the doctoral program at Brown. I won't even have to teach.

By the time I arrive in Providence, I'm sort of a hippie. I'm against the war in Vietnam, against consumer culture and in favor of peace, drugs and rock 'n roll. But I also admire rational thought, loathe astrology and plan to get a doctorate.

I'm certainly a fashion hippie (except for class). I like soft old jeans or hip-hugging bell bottoms and clinging T-shirts or flowing gauzy shifts. I have a mirrored, embroidered Indian vest that I wear a lot, sometimes over nothing. I believe in free love, and I'm on the pill.

After a summer apart, Stan and I are seeing each other again when I'm in New York, but neither of us has demanded or vowed exclusivity, and most of the time, I'm in Providence. I always prefer dating boys who get high; in general, I'm drawn to the radical types. Perhaps because my own life as a graduate student is safe, even circumscribed, rebellious guys attract me, especially those with charisma. Doug is an undergraduate student leader with dark curls and burning blue eyes. We go to bed one night and talk until the room gets light. As a political activist, he doesn't possess any pot of his own because of the general belief that the pigs will imprison radicals by busting them for grass, but he's happy to smoke whatever I might bring. One night we smoke pot and start talking about acid and how it makes you experience things differently. I'm relating an incident about a vending machine when I was high on LSD. Doug gives me an startled look. "What is it?" I ask.

"Go on."

I suddenly realize that this story about the vending machine did not happen to me but to somebody else. But to whom? I falter.

"What happened next?" Doug asks.

"Well, the machine spits out the pack of crackers, and it goes, thunk-thunk, and I think the machine just said, 'Thank you.'"

And now I know whose story this really is, just *one* second before Doug cries out, "My God, the exact same thing happened to me!"

At this point, I feel it is incumbent upon me to express astonishment and delight to match his own: how strange it is that *we both had the same experience* on separate LSD trips in our past.

After two years of classes and several "last affairs," I finish my course-work at Brown and move in with Stan. I am eager to have children and want him for the father; we agree to marry in December. Do I force the issue? Perhaps. I want to get married while in the first glow of bliss, not after years of cohabitation. But I do give Stan a choice: if he thinks December's too soon, that's fine: I'll just move into my own place. This is actually an option: a girl with little money can get her own apartment in Manhattan. But it never happens: not wanting me to date other men (for which "getting my own apartment" is code), he agrees to a December wedding, and I move in with him.

37
Teen

It's 1963, the summer before college, and I prepare for smoking pot by smoking cigarettes. Everything I have read about "marihuana"—spelling it with an "h" makes it seem heavier and more exotic—tells me it's the drug for me, but first I'll have to learn how to inhale.

Much has changed since the year before, when Paula, a girl in our class, is rumored to have gone to a pot party. My reaction: deep shock—what an idiot to risk insanity and addiction! Since then, the culture, or the counter-culture, has changed, and now at 16, I am very keen to try pot, and I want to be prepared for my initiation. I'm a camp counselor, and every night after lights out, I go the porch of my cabin and smoke a Newport. It's not easy on my throat, but after some practice, I'm able to smoke the whole thing without coughing. My evening cigarette leaves me dizzy and lightheaded, a state I enjoy. I stumble into the bunkhouse, giggling. It seems I'm getting high from tobacco, and I'm sure pot will be even better.

For ten years, until my first pregnancy (when I quit

cigarettes for good), I smoke two or three tobacco cigarettes a day. I love the feeling of smoke moving down my throat, I relish the bite to the lungs. Today, I sometimes smoke pot more for the smoking part than because I want to get high. Vaporizers are not for me.

I start going to Brooklyn College, a dozen subway stops away, but my first boyfriend that year is someone from the neighborhood, a handsome young Irishman with a chipped front tooth. I don't remember how we meet: he probably just says hello to me on Prospect Park West. Myles carries a spiral notebook imprinted "Columbia University" and says he takes classes there. He seems to be the special friend of Martin, a flamboyantly elegant man who owns a mansion on the Park and wears a long black coat with Persian lamb lapels. Are Martin and Myles lovers? But how homosexual can Myles be, I ask myself, if he's so obviously pursuing me? At Christmas, he showers my whole family with presents: an exquisite wooden marionette for my younger sister, a white wide-woven sweater for my mother, a woolen cap for my stepfather, many gifts for me. When we walk in the snow in Prospect Park, he roguishly dashes behind a tree to bring out a bottle of Scotch he has stashed away there. I shake my head; I don't want any. Myles is gallant and dashing and fun and probably alcoholic.

We kiss until my knees are weak, but it doesn't go further than that. I'm living at home and Myles seems to be living with Martin. He's vague on that point.

Not coming from a family that drinks much, only when Myles enters my life do I smell alcohol on anybody's breath.

I think it smells rather nice, much preferable to the other smells a breath can carry: old smoke, dyspepsia, cheap lipstick, decay. Nonetheless, drinking doesn't hold any allure for me: I've had wine at the family dinner table for several years, so it isn't mysterious, and getting drunk is, I think, something for immature frat boys.

One night, Myles unexpectedly produces two joints. It's a cold night, and we smoke the joints outdoors. He smokes one and I smoke the other; we don't pass them back and forth, as we aren't aware this is the etiquette.

"I don't feel anything," I say.

He says, "You will."

We go into a bar. At this time, the drinking age is 18; Myles is, or says he is, 21 (he looks older), and I've just turned 17. When questioned about my age, I unbutton my coat and that seems to do the trick. Now we sit at the bar and Myles drinks Scotch and I drink a coke, and there's a faint buzzing in my elbows. And suddenly, strangely, I'm very hungry. Laughter floats out of my ears at this realization, for I've already had dinner. This is all incredibly funny, and I start explaining to Myles as best I can between great gusts of laughter.

"Right, you don't feel it," he says, occasioning another gale of mirth.

"Do you think we could get any food here?" I finally gasp. Nothing is more important to me now: there's a vast empty cavern underneath my throat.

"Sure," he says. He orders a couple of burgers.

My hamburger arrives on a white paper plate. I bring the

burger to my mouth and take a bite, and it's the very best hamburger I've ever had. It is crisp on the edges but plump and juicy inside, and the bun is beautifully bland, exquisitely puffy, perfectly complementing the juicy treasure it encloses. I ask Myles. "How did you know this bar had such great food?"

I tell the bartender, "This is the most wonderful hamburger I've ever had."

He looks at me, baffled and hostile, as if I'm mocking him.

"It is," I insist. "It really is."

I can no longer doubt that I'm high.

Addicts, says writer Ann Marlowe, are often in "mourning for the irrecoverable glories of the first time." So true, so true! Pot may have gotten stronger now, but I'm no longer getting nearly as high as during that first year of pot-smoking as a college freshman.

"Did you like getting high?" Myles asks after that first time as he kisses me goodnight at my front door.

"Oh, yes."

"I knew you would," he says.

You and me both.

The next afternoon, while I'm away in class, there's a furious knocking at our front door. My mother glances out and opens the door to…Martin. She tells me later what ensues. Martin's gotten his credit card bill with charges for the gifts Myles bought us for Christmas, and he's demanding the return of all the presents. Martin declaims, "While Myles, or should I say *Romeo*, was courting your daughter, he was acting like a common thief!" My mother gives him back the marionette and the sweater; the other gifts have been used and cannot be returned. Martin leaves, somewhat mollified.

When I come home, my mother says, again, "I don't think Myles is the right boy for you." I'm starting to think she's right. There's something dicey about his whole situation. Myles doesn't come around for a while, probably ashamed about the presents, and I start dating other people.

A few years later, when I'm living in Providence, Myles drops by the Brooklyn brownstone with two tabs of LSD. I'm not home, my mother isn't home, but my new stepfather, Brian, invites him in. Brian and Myles end up taking acid together. Then they walk all over Prospect Park, talking until the sun comes up. Who knew they had so much in common?

The next time I smoke pot isn't nearly as pleasant as that first time with Myles. I'm at Celia's house one afternoon after class. Her best friend from high school, Sherry, is there. So is Celia's boyfriend (Celia always has a boyfriend) and a few other people (though not, alas, her brother Michael). Soon a joint is making the rounds, and I get very stoned, very fast. It is, after all, only my second time. Celia and her boyfriend go off to her bedroom, and I am lost among these strangers. But Sherry is there, with her long, dark, wavy hair, and as if drawn by silk ribbons, I cross the room to sit by her side on the couch. I ask what Celia was like at 12 and 13, but Sherry closes her eyes. She doesn't want to talk.

Why not? Doesn't she like me? Is it because now I'm Celia's best friend? I see that I could be close to Sherry if only she'd let me. There's a bond between us that goes well beyond

Celia: we are so similar! Sherry gets off the couch and walks to the kitchen. I follow her.

She turns and demands, "Why are you following me?"

I say, "We could be so close!"

She looks at me, baffled. "I don't know what you're talking about."

"We're so alike."

"We are?" She tosses her hair back.

I'm less sure of myself now, but I say. "Yes, we are."

"Look," says Sherry, "Just go away, okay?"

And she goes into the bathroom. I can't follow her there, so I wait outside. She'll change her mind.

The toilet flushes, and Sherry emerges. When she sees me, she says in disgust, "Are you still here?"

"Just give me a chance," I beg. I cringe at how slavish I sound.

"You're giving me the creeps," says Sherry. "Get lost. I mean it." She turns on her heel and leaves the room.

I'm devastated. My soul has been sucker-punched. It feels like I've lost the only friend I've ever had. Tears well in my eyes as I make my way to the closet and get my coat. Maybe if she sees me *in my coat* she'll change her mind, but though I linger in the foyer, Sherry's gone back with the others.

The subway stop is several blocks away, and by the time I reach the station, I've come down enough to see how wrong I was with Sherry. Somehow, getting high opened an emotional spigot, and all that feeling poured out over Sherry, a hapless bystander. Maybe she was high, too, and my attention only made her paranoid.

Nonetheless, for the whole train ride home I brood about the rejection.

It's the first of many rejections by women. In the 50 years since Sherry pushes me away, women end up hurting me more than men. (I say this even though Stan abruptly left me after a long marriage.) Friendships suddenly die. Overtures are not returned. I realize that if I don't contact someone I've known for five years, I'll never see her again, so once more I make the call. This is a recurrent theme in my life. I don't know why I suffer so much with women when I get along so well with men—or is it perhaps *because* I get along so well with men? Perhaps I'm altogether more tolerant of men and nicer to them because there's some chance, no matter how remote, that they might bring me ecstasy. Is that what's going on in my limbic brain?

In the spring of my freshman year at college, there are an odd number of people in my lab class for non-science majors, so while most students are paired up, there's one group of three leftover: me and two cute guys, Charles, tall and dark, and Lenny, mid-height, with a flag of silken blond hair. We three become lab partners, to my delight. I wear my best sweaters on lab days. Soon, I'm going out with each of my lab partners, because it's perfectly fine to go out with more than one person unless you're pinned or engaged. I envy Fitzgerald's heroines who sometimes have three dates with three different men in the course of one day.

(A few years later, one of my friends admits to making

love with three men in a single day, during that brief historical moment after the pill and before herpes.)

After a couple of weeks, I stop seeing Charles and concentrate on Lenny, the one with the silken hair. Lenny has a girlfriend at a college out of state, and that may be why we never get too close. Or perhaps it's because of what he once says. One night, I am lying in his arms, with my clothes on (for I am still a virgin), and I make some remark. Then he suddenly sighs, "Oh, Cathy, you're so much smarter than me!"

"I am?" I have never considered this, one way or another, but as soon as he says it, I know that it's true, and I can never look at him the same way again.

As it happens, in later life, he becomes a famous radio personality in San Francisco. Even before Facebook, we meet up again and collaborate on a radio script. His golden hair has gone, he's entirely bald, but I'm happy to learn he's still a doper.

Lenny figures large in my development as a pothead, because one night in 1964 he gives me half a film can of clean, green grass and a couple of papers, so I can get stoned by myself. Will I be paranoid, with no one around to talk me down if I'm bumming? Will I tunnel into myself, learning what lies beneath, or will I just go to sleep? What will it be like, getting high alone?

I find out the next day: I smoke in my room then go downstairs. The back garden is pulsing with sunlight and bees; puffy white clouds ride the sky. I lie on a lawn chair and angle my face to the beautiful sun. I close my eyes. My elbows are tingling, and my throat is tender with joy.

38
The Red Pill

When I tell people that my marijuana memoir reaches back into my early childhood, they say surely I wasn't smoking pot then—and of course they're right. But doesn't personality assert itself from the beginning? Don't early memories prophesy future temperament? Don't they provide clues to the riddle of identity?

Given when I am born and where I grow up, and given my early interest in sensation and altering my perceptions, being a pothead is my destiny, my fate. Long before I know about getting high, I'm getting ready.

I'm a very sensuous child and a very happy one. Until I'm about ten, I sometimes think I'm the happiest little girl in the world. I know that my mother's the most beautiful woman in the world, and in my very first memory, I am in my crib, at age two, and she enters the darkened room and comes to my side She is glittering and radiant, in a low-cut red dress and a pearl necklace, about to leave for an evening out with my father. She kisses me goodnight, then gives me a beige rubber doll with painted blue eyes and molded rubber curls. I am overjoyed, dazzled by the gift. I don't even hear my mother leave the room, I am so enraptured with the doll.

I like to revisit the memory because of the joy it contains. Perhaps for someone morose this could be counted as a sad memory, with my mother abandoning me for a time on the town, offering a cheap rubber doll as consolation. But my disposition is sunny: the memory is wonderful. Perhaps I will always tend to remember the good rather than the bad.

My second memory is so intimate that only my decision to be ruthlessly honest impels me to share it here. As with the first memory, it can be viewed in two ways. I am now about three, living in Paris with my parents, and attending a *maternelle* or nursery school. The girls wear pale checked *tabliers* or smocks that button up the back. One sunny day, I'm outside in the yard, leaning against the wall with my knees up, my *tablier* sliding down my raised thighs. It seems a good moment to investigate my panties and what lies beneath. I am moving a finger back and forth in there and am surprised by the tiny sticky sound of my labia: *tsst, tsst.* The sun is full on my face and I close my eyes in concentration and try to make the sound again. I am just so curious about that sound when—a nursery school teacher grabs my arm and pulls me up. "What are you doing?" she demands. "*Tu n'as pas honte?*" That means, "Aren't you ashamed?"

I am indeed ashamed—because I don't know why I should be ashamed. I am genuinely puzzled. Is it something about the *tsst, tsst* sound? The sun on my face with my eyes closed? Perhaps if I were French and not American, I would know why I should be ashamed. The teacher drags me to a little sink and has me wash my hands.

This memory should be utterly humiliating, yet, honestly, it doesn't feel like that. Instead, it leaves me feeling great tenderness toward this younger, innocent self who just can't fathom what she's done wrong. She's gotten no special feelings from her hand: she just wanted to reproduce the funny little sound. For a sadder person, an incident like this might prove traumatic, undermining sexual pleasure for years. But when I think about it now, the feeling is still of bewilderment, not shame, and the sun is shining on my face. My recorder of memories, my interpreter of experience, must select for the good and the happy. It's pure luck that I have such a sanguine inner scribe.

Throughout my childhood, I am fascinated by ways I can alter my consciousness. There's getting dizzy, easily achieved, but somehow more satisfying when you do it with somebody else. When I'm with another child, I'm always the one to suggest, "Let's spin round and round!" I like how when you stop turning, the room arcs back and forth and the floor heaves upward. I like the disorientation, which often makes me topple. I don't mind because I don't have far to fall.

When I'm about six, I start to fuzz. That's what I call it to myself, for I don't tell anyone about it. That's a great thing about fuzzing: no one knows I can do it, and no one knows when I do it. It's terrific in class, when I'm bored. I simply unfocus my eyes so the classroom gets blurry and I feel like

I'm floating. I'm detached from the world and at peace. I can't maintain the state for long, but it always refreshes me, like a secret little vacation into the void.

Sometimes I wonder if other kids fuzz, but I don't ever ask them. They might think I was weird.

They would certainly think I was weird if I told them something else I do in class when I'm bored. (I'm often bored because on my own I read the text books during the first two weeks of school, and after that it's all repetition.) So when the teacher's droning on about something I already know, I sometimes position my upper arm over the back of my chair in such a way that I cut off my circulation. I stay like that until my arm and hand feel "white and thin." I can't really put it into words, I just wait until the time is right. Then I get my reward. I lift my arm from the chair and let it dangle down, and a hot whoosh goes down my arm, which I call "the blood rush." I'm a fool for this sensation and other bodily enjoyments.

When my father gives me a cuckoo clock, I tie a white pillow feather to the pendulum so that it will stroke my wrist. This turns out not to be nearly as good as having someone else use the feather on my wrist. I am learning that the stimulus has to keep changing for it to be good, and that uncertainty heightens sensation. The mechanical feather is a bore.

On sleepover dates, I'm always the one who says, "Let's stroke each other's backs!" Pajama tops are immediately hiked up; no one ever refuses. I always try to go first with the stroking, so that when my back is stroked, I don't have any work to do and can just drift off into sleep. Writing on each other's backs with our fingertips is another suggestion I sometimes make: "Write a word on my back—no, write a sentence!"

At seven, I invent an odd little game I call "going to sleep." I say I've discovered that when somebody strokes my arms it always makes me drowsy, and I beg them not to do it. How can they resist? When I'm finally "asleep," I let the girl or boy do mildly mischievous things to me: line up toy cars along my back or tie my shoelaces together. (With my duller friends, I have to suggest what they might do when I finally go to sleep.) The point of this game, of course, is getting stroked.

Perhaps all children are as primed for pleasure as I am, but in my case there has been no counterforce: no throttle to the hedonistic engine. In my family of atheists, the primacy of happiness is a given, and to a child there's not much distinction between happiness and pleasure. It's a pleasure to feel the sun on my face, and most of my happiest moments occur in the sun. As a Greenwich Village girl, I always walk on the sunny side of the street, and when I skate in Washington Square Park, it's always in the sun. The rays make me feel not only warm but joyful.

By now, my parents are divorced, and my mother has married Antoine, a Belgian mechanical engineer of great vitality and charm who spent his adolescence in Cuba. He likes to challenge established opinions and takes pride in his originality of outlook. I like him at once because he's as playful as a boy. At our first meeting, I am walking in the park with my mother when he jumps out from behind a tree and asks me to play hide-and-seek. He tells me funny stories in French. He gives me an erector set, and I dutifully try to interest myself in it for his sake.

He seems to like me as much as I like him, and once he even tells me I'm one of the five people he respects most in all the world. Respects! What eight-year-old child ever hears that? I try to be worthy and interesting.

He and my mother have an active social life. At least once a week, they go to or give a dinner party, their friends trooping up the four flights of stairs to our small apartment. Just before every gathering, Antoine and my mother confer about repartee. What will they talk about at the party? What subjects will prompt the most interesting conversation or reveal new dimensions in their friends? My mother spends more time discussing repartee than she does getting dressed and made-up. This bit of pre-party planning they call "prepartee." One night when I'm ten, Antoine offers up the red pill as a subject for repartee. He says, "If a red pill could make people happy, would you take it?"

"Certainly not!" says my mother. "That would be false and artificial."

"So what? Just because something's artificial doesn't mean it's bad."

"But happiness should derive from something else, like accomplishing a goal or being with a friend."

"Why?" asks Antoine.

"That's just how it works," says my mother. "Besides, I wouldn't take the red pill because I'd be worried about the side effects."

"There aren't any side effects from the red pill."

"All drugs have side effects."

"This is a hypothetical drug," says Antoine. "It has no side effects."

"Well, it will make good repartee," admits my mother, "but I still think it's a bad idea."

"Don't be so conventional! I see nothing wrong with taking the red pill. It's a really interesting concept."

"Shhh," says my mother. "*Pas devant la petite.*"

After my two years in Paris, I can certainly understand the phrase "Not in front of the little one," as she knows very well, and I don't see why this intriguing conversation should suddenly cease.

Antoine agrees with me. "Let's ask Cathy!" he says, though my mother is frowning and shaking her head. "Cathy, darling. Supposing there was a red pill you could take that would make you feel wonderful. Would you take it?"

His eyes are wide, he's truly interested in my response. And I can make him proud of me just by telling him the truth.

It seems so obvious to me.

I say, "Of course I would!"

THE END

A NOTE ABOUT NAMES

I have given everyone who appears in this book the chance to choose a pseudonym, and I'm disheartened to report that most people have taken that option.

ABOUT THE AUTHOR

Catherine Hiller is the author of six novels: *Cybill Unbound,
The Feud, The Adventures of Sid Sawyer, California Time, 17
Morton Street, An Old Friend from High School,* and a short
story collection, *Skin: Sensual Tales.* She has also written two
children's books, *Argentaybee and the Boonie* and *Abracatabby.*
Her Substack is The Pleasure Principle. She is the co-producer
of two hour-long documentary films: *Do Not Enter: The Visa
War Against Ideas* and *Paul Bowles: The Complete Outsider.*

Catherine Hiller has a BA, *summa cum laude,* from Brooklyn
College and a PhD from Brown University. She lives with her
husband and their dog in Mamaroneck and Sag Harbor, New York.

She has smoked marijuana almost every day for the past
sixty years.